Wheels of Light

A STUDY OF THE CHAKRAS

Wheels of Light

A STUDY OF THE CHAKRAS

by
Rosalyn L. Bruyere

edited by
Jeanne Farrens

Bon Productions
Sierra Madre, California

For additional copies of this book contact:

Bon Productions
701 First Ave, Suite 307
Arcadia, CA 91006

ISBN Number: 0-923808-01-9
Library of Congress Catalog Card Number: 88-68111

DEDICATION

To all the students of seventeen years
who asked, "What's an aura?"
To all my teachers, the kind elders who said,
"You're all right, kid, but you sure are slow",
And in loving memory of Hugh Blake,
who supported this work even in passing.

PERMISSIONS

The publisher wishes to thank the following for permission to reprint selections and illustrations in this book. Any inadvertent omission will be corrected in future printings upon notification of the publisher:

Valerie V. Hunt EdD. for material from *Project Report: A Study of Structural Integration From Neuromuscular, Energy Field and Emotional Approaches.*

Harper & Row, New York, N.Y. for material from *The Great Initiates* by Edward Schure.

Harper & Row, San Francisco, CA for material from *Mystery Religions in the Ancient World* by Joscelyn Godwin.

Lucis Publishing Company, New York, N.Y. for material from *The Rays And Initiations* by Alice Bailey.

The Philosophical Research Society, Los Angeles, CA for material from *The Secret Teachings of All Ages* by Manley P. Hall.

State University of New York, Albany, N.Y. for material from *Ancient Wisdom and Modern Science,* edited by Stanislav Grof, M.D.

The Theosophical Publishing House, Wheaton, IL for material from *Talks on the Path To Occultism* by Annie Besant and C.W. Leadbeater.

The Theosophical Publishing House, Wheaton IL for material from *Theories of the Chakras* by Hiroshi Motoyama.

Penguin Books, New York, N.Y. for illustrations from *Book of the Hopi* by Frank Waters with drawings and source materials recorded by Oswald White Bear Fredericks.

Timeless Books, Porthill, ID for illustrations from *Kundalini Yoga for the West* by Swami Sivananda Radha.

Wheelwright Museum of the American Indian, Santa Fe, N.M. for illustrations from *Navaho Figurines Called Dolls* by Roger Kelly, R.W. Lang and Harry Walters.

ACKNOWLEDGMENTS

There are many whose talents, efforts and generosity have contributed to the creation of this book. From its inception to its completion, I have been fortunate to have been assisted by the kind and dedicated support of those many who gave so graciously and lovingly.

I am grateful to Dr. Valerie Hunt for her inspiration, for providing me with the first opportunity to have my personal experience of the chakras tested and corroborated scientifically and for her kind permission to include results of that research in the text and Appendix of this volume; Lyle Brady for his critical evaluation and valuable suggestions; and Terry Oleson for his support. I wish to thank Gloria Orenstein and Karen Segal for their astute observations and critques and for sharing their scholarship with me; Orville McKinley, M.D. for contributing his knowledge of Navaho ceremony and teachings; Maria Bauer Hall for sharing her convictions and the insights of work which has spanned nearly half a century; Grace Fogg at ARE, Michael King at the Theosophical Publishing House and Rebecca Lang at the Liverpool Museum for their kind and prompt assistance; and Jaime Dunaway for his critical eye and enthusiastic encouragement.

I also gratefully acknowledge Charlotte Kaiser for her drawings, and Debbie West and Paulette Kelly for their willingness to do whatever was needed to prepare this manuscript for publication. I am grateful to my researchers, Stephanie Roth, Shelby Hammit and Jeanne Farrens, for their long hours and excellent abilities; to Kristen McCall, who cheerfully and tirelessly transcribed over 3,000 pages of lecture material; and to Ken Weintrub for generously assisting me to hear my words as others will when they read this book. I wish to further express my gratitude to Robert E. Williams for his time and beautiful photographic contributions; my deep appreciation to Susan Rothschild, who can work miracles with light and a camera; and grateful acknowledgment to Karen Haskin for her generosity, her remarkable talent and her exquisite illustrations. I am profoundly grateful to Margie M. Smith for her computer drawings, her technical assistance and, most especially, for having traveled the path before me and for possessing the expertise to have brought this book to publication.

I extend heartfelt appreciation to my editorial staff, Maria Bartolotta, Susan Brown and Jeanne Farrens for their dedication, talents and generosity and sincerest gratitude to them for their continued support, affection and friendship. I would like especially to acknowledge Jeanne Farrens, for her love of both language and healing, and whose encouragement and commitment, more than that of any other, assisted me in completing this work. Finally, to those who lovingly supported me throughout this project, and to all who patiently waited for this book, thank you.

TABLE
of
CONTENTS

PART TWO—THE FIRST CHAKRA

—PART ONE—

WHEELS OF LIGHT

Chapter One

THEORY AND TERMS

My Initiation

Chakras, as well as auras and electromagnetic fields, are as old as the earth itself. As we explore the chakras, as we voyage into the complexities of auric and electromagnetic fields and corresponding energy exchanges, it is important for us to view our journey not as revolutionary, but rather as very traditional. The chakra system, in fact, is a part of the ancient and lost mysteries. It is an energy system which keeps body and mind alive and healthy, and which may in actuality create them. The seven chakras are who and what we are, what we feel and how we think and change. They are how we express ourselves and how we create. Although as Westerners, we have no cognitive awareness of its energies, the chakra system is precisely the means by which we gain awareness. It is how we experience life, how we perceive reality and how we relate to self, others and the world. It is life itself. And finally, the chakra system is how we find our way back to the most ancient Mystery of all—God, the Oneness, the Omniscient.

In my seventeen years of practice as a healer and a teacher of healing, I have collected a great amount of information about the chakra system. Different religious traditions call these energy centers different things. The word most commonly used is *chakra* from the Sanskrit word meaning "wheel of light". The majority of what I know about the chakra system has come directly from my experience as a healer and aura reader: putting "energy"[1] into a body and watching its movement. I observed that adding energy to one part of the body reveals how the body uses energy, which in turn discloses the overall state of health. I watched people think. I watched them feel. I saw that these "patterns" corresponded to their disease. From this experience I learned that we can suppress information in the body or in the chakra system, but we can never eliminate it. We can alter that information by the way we move or the way we think. Even if we make a slight change in behavior, it precipitates change in every other aspect of our lives.

These observations could have remained subjective, but very early in my career I was given the fortunate and unique opportunity to have the process observed in a formal research environment. At the conclusion of that research my personal experience of the nature of the chakra system had been validated, and I resolved ever after to always seek the science within the spiritual and the spiritual within science.

I was specifically not interested in anything esoteric as a young person. I had a psychic grandmother and great-grandmother with whom I spent many hours as a child. In fact I was even taught to see auras on plants as a youth, although I did not remember that experience at all until after I began my own study of healing and mediumship. The esoteric had always been around me, but I never paid any attention to it.

Then I married and had children who

---

[1]   Although in scientific terminology, energy is strictly defined as "the capacity for doing work", I use it throughout this text to denote the various frequencies and magnitude of oscillations within a dynamic electromagnetic field. Cf. p 20 for a more thorough explanation. Also see Fig. 3.8, p. 63.

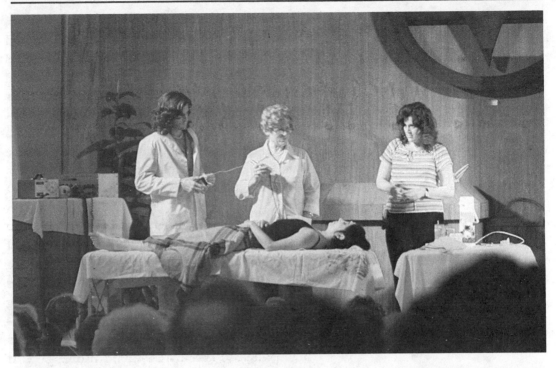

began to speak about the "colored fuzz" around people. They were seeing auras. Their "sight" restimulated my own. In order to raise them responsibly I was forced to seek out the teachers who could help me make sense of our experiences. My studies not only helped me make sense of those experiences but introduced me to their practical applications. I was taught rudimentary healing techniques, which I sometimes practiced on my friends. I had no intention of becoming a healer, but I became one as the people I "treated" began to feel better and talk about it.

I also developed a reputation as an aura reader since when people came to me I would explain what an aura was and how I saw their disease. One day a woman phoned, identifying herself as a healer. She asked if she could bring a client to my home and requested me to tell her what I saw in the aura of the client as she worked. I was

Fig. 1.1. REVIEWING THE ROLF STUDY. Standing from left to right: Dr. Hunt's assistant, Dr. Valerie Hunt, and Rosalyn Bruyere. Emilie Conrad Dáoud is lying on the table.

completely unprepared for what transpired. Rather than laying-on-of-hands which I had been taught, Emilie Conrad Dáoud used chanting and dancing in a very involved process. At the end of that process I told her what I had seen aurically. She then took that information to Dr. Valerie Hunt at UCLA who was researching the same process from the viewpoint of a kinesiologist. Eventually I was asked to work in collaboration with both of them.

The research we did was significant on more than one level. It was perhaps the first attempt made in our country to examine an electrical manifestation, a magnetic field phenomenon as connected to the healing process. Prior to that time, laying-on-of-hands healing had been viewed as a psychological, not an energetic process. Our research was important in that it was a meaningful attempt to correlate the body's natural frequency ranges (which had already been monitored by kinesiology) with the spiritual world. Dr. Hunt had received a grant to study Structural Integration (or rolfing as it is commonly called), and that became part of the research project.[2] The study concluded that rolfing made a lasting change on the body's energy. The research also illustrated that "spiritual energy" was real energy, discernible and measurable as frequencies in the body. This was a tremendous breakthrough in the field of science.

Because of the impact of that research, I developed a reputation and a legitimacy beyond my years of experience. Subsequently I was given a series of opportunities that I otherwise might not have been given. The first of these introduced me to the Native American world. I was asked to

[2]   Valerie V. Hunt, *Project Report: A Study of Structural Integration from Neuromuscular, Energy Field, and Emotional Approaches*, Boulder, Colorado: Rolf Institute of Structural Integration, 1977. This research will hereafter be referred to in the text as the Rolf Study.

heal one of the Hopi tribal elders, Grandfather David Monongya. He was in Los Angeles to raise consciousness regarding the strip mining at Big Mountain, site of one of the first conflicts over the Hopi/Navajo tribal land. Grandfather David had cataracts. I laid hands on his body and very quickly moved to his head and laid hands on his eyes. He seemed to know exactly what I was doing. About the time I was actually beginning to accomplish something that I felt was healing, he said, "Oh, I see much better now. Please sit down." Of course I had not healed him, and in a manner of speaking, as it turned out, I ended up receiving a healing from him. He called to two or three other people in the house, and we listened for five hours as he related the Hopi prophecy. I was stunned by the similarities between the story of the Apocalypse in Revelations and the predictions for the "end time" in Hopi.

I began to compare different cultures with different religious traditions as a way of finding other similarities in their teachings and sacred mysteries. The more I studied, the more I found varied cultural references to the chakra system. Shortly after my meeting with Grandfather David, I made a journey to the Holy Land. There I found that the chakra system as I knew and understood it meant something different once I was removed from my own culture and cultural heritage. I discovered that the light—the aura—and the meaning of the auric colors often differed from culture to culture. In Western society, people tend to think in yellow, daydream in blue, change in green and get angry in red. While this tendency is not absolute, it is generally consistent. In traveling 600 miles up the Egyptian Nile I never saw blue or yellow in the auras of Islamic people; I also noticed that

Fig. 1.2. *THE ESSENCE OF HOPI PROPHECY. See pages 8-10.*

The Essence of Hopi Prophecy

The entire Hopi prophecy usually takes many days to tell, and many lifetimes to fully understand. This is a short summary of essential points.

The Balance of Life

As caretakers of life we affect the balance of nature to such a degree that our own actions determine whether the great cycles of nature bring prosperity or disaster. Our present world is the unfoldment of a pattern we set in motion.

Our divergence from the natural balance is traced to a point preceding the existence of our present physical form. Once we were able to appear and disappear at will, but through our own arrogance we took our procreative powers for granted and neglected the plan of the creator. As a consequence we became stuck in our physical form, dominated by a continual struggle between our left and right sides, the left being wise but clumsy, and the right being clever and powerful but unwise, forgetful of our original purpose.

The Cycle of Worlds

This suicidal split was to govern the entire course of our history through world after world. As life resources diminished in accord with the cycles of nature, we would try to better our situation through our own inventions, believing that any mistakes could be corrected through further inventions. In our cleverness, most of us would lose sight of our original purpose, become involved in a world of our own design, and ultimately oppose the order of the universe itself, becoming the mindless enemy of the few who would still hold the key to survival.

In several previous worlds the majority have advanced their technology in this way, even beyond what we know today. The consequent violations against nature and fellow humans caused severe imbalances which were resolved in the form of war, social disintegration and natural catastrophe.

As each world reached the brink of annihilation, there remained a small minority who had managed to live in nearly complete accord with the infinite plan, as implied in the name, Hopi. Toward the final stages they would find themselves beset with signs of disintegration within, as well as enticing offers and severe threats from without, aimed toward forcing them to join the rest of the world.

Our Present World

Our common ancestors were among the small group who miraculously emerged from the last world as it reached its destruction, though they too were tainted with corruption. The seeds of the crisis we face today were brought with us when we first set foot in this world.

Upon reaching our present world, our ancestors set out on a long migration to meet the Great Spirit in the form of **Maasauu**, the caretaker of this land and all that lives upon it. They followed a special pattern, however a very serious omen made a separate journey necessary, in order to balance the extreme disorder anticipated for the later days.

The True White Brother

A Hopi of light complexion now known as the "true white brother", left the group and travelled in the direction of the rising sun, taking with him a stone tablet which matches a similar tablet held by one of those who went on to meet Maasauu at a place called Oraibi, where the present Hopi villages were established according to his instruction.

The Hopi anticipated the arrival of a race of light-skinned people from the east, predicting many of their inventions, which would serve as signs indicating certain stages of the unfoldment of the pattern the Hopi had studied from antiquity. It was clearly foreseen that the visitors, in their cleverness, might lose sight of their original purpose, in which case they would be very dangerous. Still the Hopi were to watch for one who has not left the spiritual path, and carries the actual stone tablet.

The Swastika and the Sun

Through countless centuries the Hopi have recalled in their cere-monies the previous worlds, our emergence to the present world, and our purpose in coming here. Periodically they have renewed their vow with Maasauu to live the simple, humble way of life he laid out for them, and to preserve the balance of nature for the sake of all living things. The knowledge of world events has been handed down in secret religious societies who keep watch as each stage unfolds.

The leaders watched especially for a series of three world-shaking events, accompanied by the ap-pearance of certain symbols that describe the primordial forces that govern all life, from the sprouting of a seed to global movements such as weather, earthquakes, migrations and wars.

The gourd rattle is a key symbol. A gourd signifies seed force. The shaking of the gourd rattle in ceremonies means the stirring of life forces. On the rattle are drawn the

ancient symbols of the swastika, showing the spirals of force sprouting from a seed in four directions, surrounded by a ring of red fire, showing the encircling penetration of the sun's warmth which causes the seed to sprout and grow.

The first two world-shaking events would involve the forces portrayed by the swastika and the sun. Out of the violence and destruction of the first, the strongest elements would emerge with still greater force to produce the second event. When the actual symbols appeared it would be clear that this stage of the prophecy was being fulfilled.

The Gourd Full of Ashes

Eventually a "gourd full of ashes" would be invented, which if dropped from the sky would boil the oceans and burn the land, causing nothing to grow there for many years. This would be the signal for a certain Hopi to bring out his teachings in order to warn the world that the third and final event would happen soon, and that it could bring an end to all life unless people correct themselves and their leaders in time.

Hopi leaders now believe the first two events were the first and second world wars, and the "gourd full of ashes" is the atomic bomb. After the bombing of Hiroshima and Nagasaki, teachings formerly kept secret were compared and released to the world. The details presented here are part of those teachings.

The Day of Purification

The final stage, called the "great day of purification" has also been described as a "mystery egg", in which the forces of the swastika and the sun, plus a third force, symbolized by the color red, culminate either in total rebirth, or total annihilation—we don't yet know which, but the choice is ours. War and natural catastrophe may be involved. The degree of violence will be determined by the degree of inequity caused among the peoples of the world and in the balance of nature. In this crisis, rich and poor will be forced to struggle as equals to survive.

That it will be very violent is now almost taken for granted among traditional Hopi, but man may still lessen the violence by correcting his treatment of nature and fellow man. Ancient spiritually-based communities, such as the Hopi, must especially be preserved and not forced to abandon their wise way of life and the natural resources they have vowed to protect.

The Fate of Mankind

The Hopi play a key role in the survival of the human race, through their vital communion with the unseen forces that hold nature in balance, as an example of a practical alternative to the suicidal man-made system, and as a fulcrum of world events. The pattern is simple, "The whole world will shake and turn red and turn against those who are hindering the Hopi."

The man-made system now destroying Hopi is deeply involved in similar violations throughout the world. The devastating reversal predicted in the prophecies is part of the natural order. If those who thrive from that system, its money and its laws, can manage to stop it from destroying Hopi, then many may be able to survive the day of purification and enter a new age of peace. But if no one is left to continue the Hopi Way, then the hope for such an age is in vain.

The forces we must face are formidable, but the only alternative is annihilation. Still the man-made system cannot be corrected by any means that requires one's will to be forced upon another, for that is the source of the problem. If people are to correct themselves and their leaders, the gulf between the two must disappear. To accomplish this one can only rely on the energy of truth itself.

This approach, which is the foundation of the Hopi way of life, is the greatest challenge a mortal can face. Few are likely to accept it. But once peace is established on this basis, and our original way of life is allowed to flourish, we will be able to use our inventive capacity wisely, to encourage rather than threaten life, and benefit everyone rather than giving advantage to a few at the expense of others. Concern for all living things will far surpass personal concerns, bringing greater happiness than could formerly be realized. Then all living things shall enjoy lasting harmony.

Written by Thomas V. Tarbet, Jr., and reviewed by a traditional messenger. Free copies of this information may be obtained from:

PLANTING STICK
ROUTE 3, BOX 78
SANTA FE, NM 87501

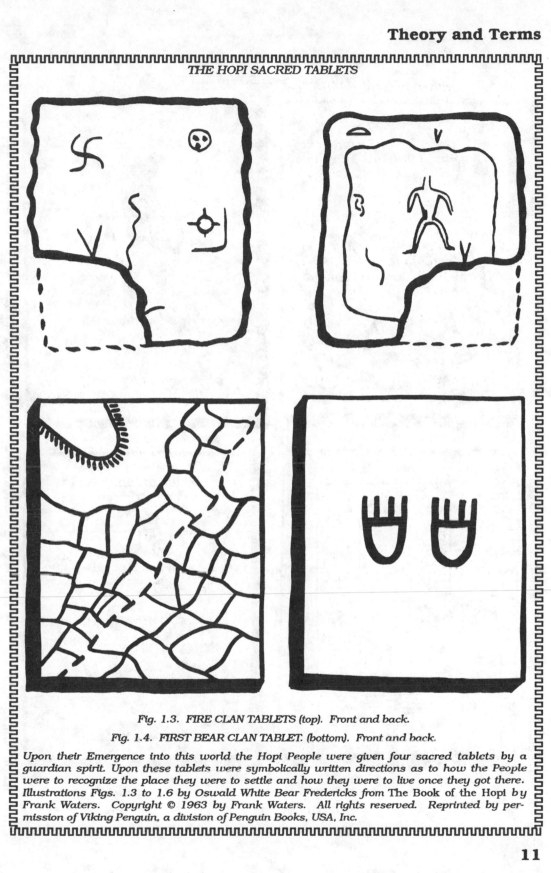

THE HOPI SACRED TABLETS

Fig. 1.3. FIRE CLAN TABLETS (top). Front and back.

Fig. 1.4. FIRST BEAR CLAN TABLET. (bottom). Front and back.

Upon their Emergence into this world the Hopi People were given four sacred tablets by a guardian spirit. Upon these tablets were symbolically written directions as to how the People were to recognize the place they were to settle and how they were to live once they got there. Illustrations Figs. 1.3 to 1.6 by Oswald White Bear Fredericks from The Book of the Hopi *by Frank Waters.* *Copyright © 1963 by Frank Waters.* *All rights reserved.* *Reprinted by permission of Viking Penguin, a division of Penguin Books, USA, Inc.*

THE HOPI SACRED TABLETS

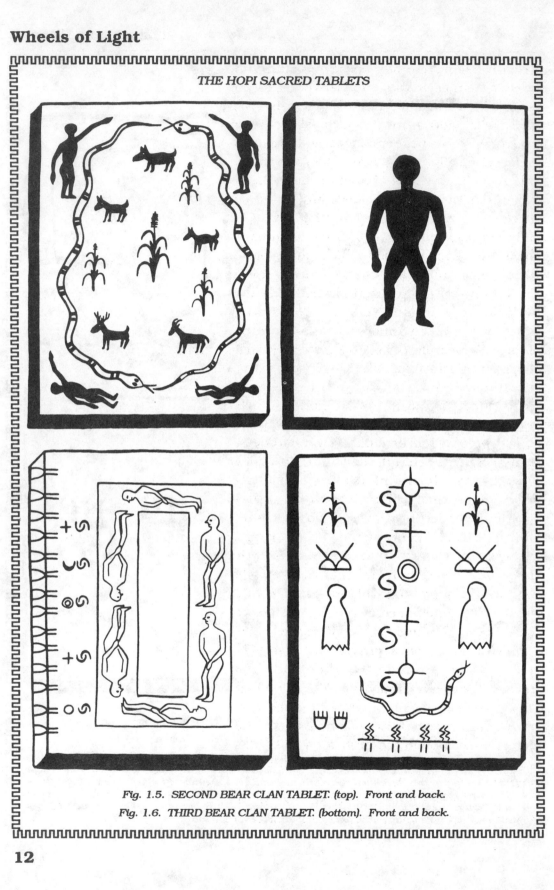

Fig. 1.5. *SECOND BEAR CLAN TABLET. (top). Front and back.*
Fig. 1.6. *THIRD BEAR CLAN TABLET. (bottom). Front and back.*

aurically their thought process seemed to closely resemble that of the Native American people whom I had observed. Once in Israel I again saw yellow auric fields, an observation which led me to believe that Israelis tend to "think" more like Europeans and Americans. From these experiences I began to comprehend why, in the Middle East, Israelis and Arabs do not seem to understand each other's way of thinking and why, on our own continent, the Native Americans and non-indigenous peoples fail to understand each other's ways. These observations led me to question whether or not the practices of different religions and particularly prayer positions change the auric colors. I especially began to wonder whether thought was something other than logic as we know it in the West.

Once I began to explore things in this way, it followed that if an entire culture's thought process was dominated by a particular chakra color, that culture would process reality through that dominant chakra. In other words, since each chakra has a particular "viewpoint", a culture would tend to "see" reality through the "eyes" of that chakra. Furthermore, because each chakra is directly related to a specific area of the body, certain positions and postures of the body would enhance the dominance of one or two colors while inhibiting others. In Islam, for instance, a Moslem bows, on a prayer rug, with his knees on the ground. He then puts his forehead (more specifically, his "third eye") on a point that is usually a design on the rug. This posture directs focus to the area around the navel and around the forehead, making the second (orange) and sixth (purple) chakras dominant.

As one chakra center becomes predominant in a given culture, that chakra

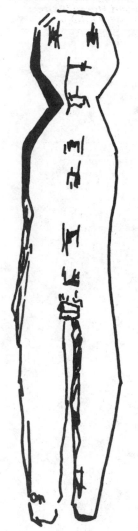

"colors" the values, assumptions and prejudices of that society. This in turn often creates a prevailing one-mindedness or dogmatism. Such narrowness of vision has often determined the characteristics of a culture and the course of an era.

As far as I can tell, Native Americans are the only people who have a natural relationship with the chakra system that has not been dogmatized. Therefore, they have not made any chakras right or wrong, good or bad, hot or cold, more important or less important. They have not had to make their world view fit that of Christianity, Judaism, Islam, Hinduism or Buddhism. Whereas these religions have evolved priesthoods that have both written in and written out various ideas over the centuries, the Native Peoples have an attitude that all the chakra centers are good, valid and important. These people, who, by their own accounts have lived here for fifteen thousand years, have had a working knowledge of the body's energy system since that time.[3] They also have maintained a tradition of practices, rituals and ceremonies that affect those energy centers.

I have been greatly influenced by the traditions and ways of these peoples. Furthermore, because of my ability to see the effect they have on us, I have been deeply moved to learn their ways and ceremonies and to include them in my work. I do not see these practices as being in conflict with anything else I know religiously. I view them as part of understanding religion. Like the Native Americans, I believe the energy field of the earth itself resonates up through our bodies, which is why I think it is natural for me to worship as a native person would. Practicing religion with the plants, the herbs

[3] Refer to Frank Waters, *Book of the Hopi*, New York: Penguin Books, 1985, pp. 9-11.

14

and the animals that exist where I am makes me more connected and more ecologically responsible to the ground upon which I live, and I find the simplicity with which one can pray with what naturally occurs around him absolutely as it should be.

The more I studied Native American culture as well as the ancient traditions of the Egyptians and Greeks, the philosophies of the Hindus and the religions of the East, the more I realized the potential value of the chakra system as a means of understanding life and energy and the symbolic relationship between them. As a young teacher of this material, I kept trying to find a textbook from which to teach. I found none. The few books available presented their own unique theories and ideas and were generally contradictory of one another. This book in many ways is an attempt to create a source that pulls those ideas together. In so doing, I had to face the fact that this material has no beginning and has no end; it is evolving, a work in progress, as is the human race.

I am writing this text primarily for Americans, mainly for students of healing. If this book serves its purpose, it will become obsolete. Those who study the chakra system will acquire an understanding of it and will then be able in their own individual ways to add to it the knowledge they accumulate through their own experience. This book is merely a foundation from which a greater structure is certain to arise.

It is my hope that those who read this book will find, as I have, support and validation for many aspects of themselves. My study of the chakra system has allowed me to develop many elements of my own being, without having to sacrifice one for the other. I have been able to embrace motherhood and

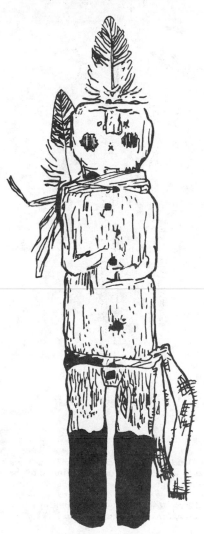

Fig. 1.8. DOLL. In this drawing, all seven chakras are indicated by the bits of stone, coral and shell inserted into the figurine. (There is one stone at the top of the head of the doll which is hard to see.) According to Dr. Orville McKinley, a Navaho physician, figurines of this sort are used in teaching medicine men and women how to diagnose conditions by feeling auras.

Drawing also courtesy of Navaho Figurines Called Dolls (figure 17, page 46, Wheelwright Museum of the American Indian Collection) by Roger E. Kelly, R. W. Lang and Harry Walters, 1972, Museum of Navajo Ceremonial Arts, Santa Fe, New Mexico.

the ministry, art and engineering; I have been allowed wholeheartedly and without conflict to live up to my resolution to pursue the spiritual in science and science in the spiritual.

In seeking the scientific in the spiritual, I have clearly been influenced by my early scientific background. I have searched for whatever validating "empirical" data I could find. Until recently, though, chakras have had little validation in the scientific world. Nevertheless, these powerful energy centers have been spinning, creating and recording their symbolic reality since the beginning of time.

In antiquity, before science and religion were divided into separate, antagonistic camps, the chakras were an integrated part of daily life. Not only were they an aspect of spiritual tradition and practice, but as a reflection of the natural laws of the greater macrocosm, they were also at the root of the ancient sciences as well. The people of antiquity (the Egyptians, Chinese, Hindus, Greeks and, in our own country, the Native Americans) knew of these phenomena, although they may have called them by different names. Furthermore, these peoples attempted to preserve and transmit this knowledge through teachings and sacred ceremony.[4] Within that ceremony one was taught to quiet bodily functions and to silence the mind long enough to observe his own internal silence wherein he could become aware of the presence, reality and power of the chakras, of the flows of energy moving through him. Then, when the Dark Ages descended upon the world, both the scientific and religious traditions of old were forced into the dark recesses of secluded rooms and secret chambers.

4   The *Bardo Thodol* or *Tibetan Book of the Dead*, the Vedic texts of the Hindus, as well as the Hermetic texts (attributed to the Egyptian god-scribe, Tehuty-Thoth) and the writings of Iamblicus, Plato, Apuleius and Proclus contain such teachings and descriptions of such ceremonies.

As each of the ancient civilizations was conquered—the Egyptian, the Chinese, the Greek, the Roman—vast libraries were burned and within the fires were consumed massive volumes of antiquarian and esoteric wisdom. It is no mistake that the period which followed was termed the Dark Ages. By the time the light shone again, science and religion had become enemies, and common knowledge of the chakra system had become an esoteric mystery.

These mysteries, however, were preserved by sacred priesthoods[5] and transmitted to select initiates throughout the ages. In our own culture the Native Americans have preserved these ideas through oral tradition. Moreover, it was prophesied by nearly every ancient culture that there would be a future time when this "lost" knowledge would be rediscovered.

> That which is a mystery shall no longer be so, and that which has been veiled will now be revealed; that which has been withdrawn will emerge into the light, and all men shall see and together they shall rejoice.[6]

That future which was prophesied has come. This new age which is dawning is the time wherein the ancient mysteries shall be once more revealed.

It has taken thousands of years, but within this century both scientists and spiritual seekers alike have once again begun to view the laws of nature and the laws of God as reflections of the same truth. It is this viewpoint which has allowed for scientific investigations into the nature of the chakra system and the aura and the relationship between them and the mind.

5   The two volume set of H.P. Blavatsky's *The Secret Doctrine*, Pasadena, California: Theosophical University Press, 1974 is a description in detail of this most ancient arcana which, according to the author, is a "Parent Doctrine, father and mother to all religions and mystical teachings." It was the "universally diffused religion of the ancient and prehistoric world." In her Introductory to Vol. I she further states that "Proofs of its diffusion, authentic records of its history, a complete chain of documents, showing its character and presence in every land, together with the teaching of all its great adepts, exist to this day in the secret crypts of libraries belonging to the Occult Fraternity." According to Marie Bauer Hall one such crypt is the Bruton Masonic Vault located in the Williamsburg, Virginia churchyard (*Foundations Unearthed*, Los Angeles, California: Veritas Press, 1974). Hall, who has spent nearly fifty years in research, also affirms the existence of a wisdom which predates any known philosophy but which has been preserved at Bruton and within other similar vaults world-wide. It is her belief that the "veil" has already begun to be lifted on this wisdom. (Editor's interview, September 23, 1986.) Blavatsky too writes of the lifting of this veil in our era: "... in the twentieth century... scholars will begin to recognize that the *Secret Doctrine* has neither been invented nor exaggerated, but, on the contrary, simply outlined; and finally, that its teachings antedate the Vedas... In Century the Twentieth some disciple more informed, and far better fitted, may be sent by the Masters of Wisdom to give final and irrefutable proofs that there exists a Science called *Gupta-Vidya*; and that, like the once-mysterious sources of the Nile, the source of all religions and philosophies now known to the world has been for many ages forgotten and lost to men, but is at last found." (*The Secret Doctrine*, Vol. 1, pp. xxvii and xxviii).

6   Alice Bailey, *The Rays and the Initiations*, Vol. V, New York: Lucis Publishing Company, 1972, p. 332. She continues, "So runs the Old Commentary when referring to the present cycle through which mankind is passing."

In fact, recent scientific studies are entertaining the theory that the chakra system, the aura (or the auric field) and the mind are all interrelated. In actuality they may be one and the same. New techniques such as Kirlian photography and biofeedback as well as recent research into the auric field, the electromagnetic field and mind-field phenomenon all point to the possibility of such a relationship. Wilder Penfield's *The Mystery of the Mind*,[7] Karl Pribram's *Languages of the Brain*,[8] Dr. Robert O. Becker's *The Body Electric*,[9] W. A. Tiller's[10] work, and the auric field research of UCLA's Dr. Valerie Hunt[11] on whose investigative team I served, all shed light on the connection between chakras, auras and the mind.[12] Similar, and in some cases, more thorough research has been in progress in the Soviet Union since the 1920's.[13] As a result of the research which has been done in both the East and the West, we now have a specific vocabulary by which the aura or the auric field—the chakra system—may be described.

Working Vocabulary

The *aura*, or *auric field*, as referred to in this book, relates to the *electromagnetic field* which emanates from all matter. People who are able to see auras often report a kind of luminous radiation surrounding an individual, usually consisting of one or sometimes several colors. This luminous radiation, which usually extends five or six inches around the body, is outside the range of our normal vision and in what is sometimes termed the realm of psychic sight. The difficulty in describing this to people who do not possess psychic or "second" sight, as it is also called, is that those of us who do

[7] Wilder Penfield, *The Mystery of the Mind*, Princeton, New Jersey: Princeton University Press, 1976.

[8] Karl Pribram, *Languages of the Brain*, New Jersey: Prentice Hall, 1971.

[9] Robert O. Becker, M.D. and Gary Selden, *The Body Electric: Electro-magnetism and the Foundation of Life*, New York: William Morrow and Company, Inc., 1985.

[10] See W. A. Tiller, "Energy Fields and the Human Body", *Frontiers of Consciousness*, ed. J. W. White, New York: Julian Press, 1974.

[11] The Rolf Study. Cf. note p. 6.

[12] Also refer to Harold Saxton Burr, *The Fields of Life: Our Links with the Universe*, New York: Ballentine, 1972. This book describes thirty years of Dr. Burr's research into life fields and contains a complete bibliography of his scientific publications. One ecstatic reviewer, Colin Wilson, suggests that Burr's book "could be just as important as *The Origin of the Species*," (quoted by Jeffrey Mishlove in *The Roots of Consciousness: Psychic Liberation Through History, Science and Experience*, New York: Random House Inc., 1975, p. 332. For its bibliography alone this book is worth having.) Also see *The Energies of Consciousness*, ed. Stanley Krippner and Daniel Rubin, New York: Gorden and Breach Science Publishers, Inc., 1975.

[13] See A. S. Presman, *Electromagnetic Fields and Life*, trans. F. L. Sinclair, ed. F. A. Brown, New York: Plenum Press, 1970. This volume is a thorough study of the Soviet work in bio-magnetics. Presman is on the biophysics faculty at Moscow University. Other noteworthy references are "Electromagnetic Fields and the Brain" by Yurij A. Kholodov in *Impact: Of Science and Society*, Vol. 24, no. 4, October, 1974. Kholodov is one of the top Soviet researchers in the area of biomagnetic interactions. *Impact* is published by UNESCO; "Biological Plasma of Human and Animal Organisms" by V.M. Inyushin, Symposium of Psychotronics, Prague, September, 1970, published by the Paraphysical Laboratory, Downton, Wilshire, England (all cited in Mishlove, op. cit.); Shiela Ostrander and Lynn Schroder, *Psychic Discoveries Behind the Iron Curtain*, Englewood Cliffs, New Jersey: Prentice Hall, 1971.

possess it see the colors of chakras and the auric field as vividly as others see the colors of clothes. The colors are red, orange, yellow, green, blue, violet, and white, with variations in shades and mixes, but all have a luminous glow that comes from the life-giving energy that is the auric field.

These auric field colors are very specifically related to the chakras. My experience indicates that each chakra has four discernible characteristics that functionally affect the aura: color, size and shape, rotation or spin, and intensity (which is a function of the "openness"[14] and thus the amount of energy that is produced by the chakra). It is out of these characteristics that the aura is generated. As a chakra spins, it produces its own electromagnetic field which combines with the fields generated by the other chakras to produce what we call the auric field. The amount of energy produced by a particular chakra (or group of chakras) determines the color that dominates the auric field. Thus, in a highly emotional state when the second chakra is dominant, the auric field of that person is predominantly orange, while one who is in a state of high creativity (utilizing the fifth chakra) will generally have an auric field that is predominantly blue.

This auric field is also related to the mind. When most of us think of the mind, we immediately think of the brain. Recently, however, science has begun to postulate that the mind is not *in* the brain.[15] Specifically, thought and memory seem to exist throughout the body, memory being logged primarily within the body's fascia or connective tissue.[16] Furthermore, thought itself can also be described as a form of energy.[17]

Energy as it is used in this book refers

[14] Although a chakra in actuality cannot be "open" or "closed", these terms are frequently used in discussions about the chakras in reference to the amount of energy which is actually being produced by any given chakra at any given time. Cf. p.66, Chapter Three.

[15] Penfield, op. cit.

[16] This was, in essence, the conclusion drawn by Wilhelm Reich based on years of observation and clinical experience. Refer to Wilhelm Reich, *The Discovery of the Orgone*, Vol. 1. New York: Orgone Institute Press, 1948. Besides Reichian therapy, other physical therapeutic techniques, among them Structural Integration or rolfing (qv), Alexander Technique (qv), and the Feldenkrais Method (qv) have as their basis the interrelationship between body and mind. For a detailed discussion of Reichian therapy refer to *Man in the Trap* by Elsworth Baker, M.D., New York: Avon, 1967. Baker is considered by many to be the most eminent Reichian therapist.

[17] See *Ancient Wisdom and Modern Science*, ed. Stanislav Grof, M.D., Albany, New York: State University of New York, 1984, Chapter 1.

19

to an electromagnetic field in the form of either *potential* or *kinetic* energy. Kinetic energy is energy in movement within either a *static* or *dynamic* electromagnetic field. A field is considered static until the intensity of either the electric or the magnetic field is varied. A dynamic electromagnetic field consists of oscillations of a specific frequency or wavelength; a more complex field may have several frequencies. In a dynamic field, the magnitude of the oscillations determines the intensity of the field, or the amount of energy being carried in the field. The frequency and wavelength determine the "color" of the propagation.[18] Thus, when we refer to the energy moving from chakra to chakra, or through the body, it is understood that this energy is being carried by moving electromagnetic fields. When we refer to "color of energy" (or, sometimes, *frequency*), we mean the color of the energy or chakra, as defined by the wavelength of electromagnetic radiation being emitted at that location, as perceived by those who have second sight.

The sum of potential and kinetic energy is always constant. The law of conservation holds that energy can neither be created nor destroyed. Thus, energy cannot be extracted from or added to an electromagnetic field without a corresponding change in the field. A *thought* then can be referred to as a potential or *static* electromagnetic field pattern. On the other hand, the thinking process represents a continally changing or *dynamic* electromagnetic field. As thought changes from a static to a dynamic field, it imparts energy to and receives energy from the thinker during the course of the thinking process. When the process ends, the resultant thought is stored (a memory) as a static electromagnetic field

[18] Propagation is a term used to describe the extension or transmission of sound waves or of electromagnetic radiation through air or water.

pattern in the auric field. Clearly the mind, the aura and the electromagnetic chakra system are inseparably interrelated.

Perhaps, as past sages believed, history is not linear but cyclical.[19] If this is so, then ancient wisdom and modern scientific thought are not as far apart in the time-space continuum as we may have once believed. In the words of Fritjof Capra:

> A dramatic change of concepts and ideas has occurred in physics during the first three decades of the century. Still being elaborated in our current theories of matter, the new concepts have profoundly changed our world view from the mechanistic thinking of Descartes and Newton to a holistic and ecological view. ... It is ... not surprising that the new vision of reality comes very close to the views of mystics of all ages and traditions and, in particular, to the views held in the spiritual traditions of India. Ten years ago, I was amazed to find the most striking parallels between modern physics and Eastern mysticism. These parallels can now be extended with equal justification to biology, psychology and other sciences. We now can say, with considerable confidence, that the ancient wisdom of the East provides the most consistent philosophical background to our modern scientific theories.[20]

Astrologically, the age of Aquarius is reputed to be the age of the common man.[21] When in the ancient world it was foretold that this age of Aquarius would be the time when

[19] This is a common belief held by most Eastern and Mystery religions. In addition, Pythagoras and Plato, themselves initiates of the mystery schools, embraced this view of history as well as the cyclical evolution of mankind. See Grof, op. cit., p. 11 and Joscelyn Godwin, *Mystery Religions in the Ancient World*, New York: Harper and Row, Publishers, Inc., 1981, pp. 72-73.

[20] Fritjof Capra in Grof, op. cit. pp. 135 and 137. Fritjof Capra, Ph.D., studied theoretical physics at the University of Vienna in Austria and has done research at numerous universities. He is presently working at the University of California at Berkeley and is the author of *The Tao of Physics* (qv.) and *The Turning Point* (qv.)

[21] In astrology the sign of Aquarius is associated with both the individual and individuality. The key word of Aquarius is "I know", and Aquarians are disseminators of knowledge. With the discovery of the natures of the outer planets, Aquarius, once thought to be ruled by Saturn, is now believed to be ruled by Uranus—the erratic revolutionary—which electrifyingly energizes the Universe. (Jim Maynard, *Celestial Influences*, Ashland, Oregon: Quicksilver Productions, 1987).

21

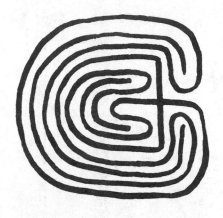

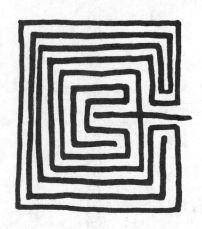

all the ancient "lost" mysteries and their importance would be revealed to the common person, a seed of hope for the future of the planet was sown. Now the season of harvest has come.

It is significant that one of the last two discovered planets, Uranus, was first sighted not by a scientist viewing the stars from an observatory on high, but by a simple curious stargazer observing the heavens through his own domestic telescope.[22] Esoteric knowledge which was lost in the flames that consumed the great library of Alexandria is being rediscovered within the laboratories of modern science. Things that were mysterious five thousand years ago in Egypt are now being taught to children in their first physics class.

"The secret mysteries of the People," foretold the Hopis a thousand years ago, "shall be made known when the sons of White men wear beads and long hair. The truth of these Sacred Ways shall be revealed when the Eagle lands on the moon."[23] Any of us who remember the Sixties and NASA's moon flights know that these events have already come to pass.

If the ideas contained within this book are difficult and challenging, it may assist us to remember that others before us were likewise challenged. Perhaps, most importantly, it would be worth our time and energy to think about what the rediscovery of these ideas could mean for us both personally and globally. These ancient, now reborn, mysteries may very well provide the kind of wisdom we need to guide us through the fears, disease and darkness of a nuclear world into a new age of hope and understanding, health and light. The very survival of the race may depend on the ability

[22] In 1781 William Herschel (1738-1822), professional musician and amateur astronomer, discovered the planet Uranus while looking through one of his homemade telescopes. Herschel became famous overnight and was soon after elected to become a fellow of the Royal Society of London and Astronomer to King George III. He eventually founded sidereal astronomy for the systematic observation of the heavens, hypothesized that nebulae are composed of stars and developed a theory of stellar evolution. (*Encyclopaedia Britannica*, Vol. 5, 1985. pp. 888-889).

[23] The words of Hopi Elder, Grandfather David Monongya, oral tradition.

of each of us to embrace new ways of thinking and being and to adopt both a traditional and revolutionary path.

It is my hope that you will view this book with a sense of exploration, as an adventure into your own personal un-discovered realms. I would also hope that at the end of the journey you will have begun to grow in health and fulfillment because you will have come closer to embracing the totality of yourself with love and understanding.

Let us begin now to unravel some of these ancient and sacred mysteries.

Chapter Two

WHEELS OF POWER

Legend of the Rainbow Warrior

The tribe that holds Second Chance Mesa sacred had at one time a great Medicine Chief who was said to see the rainbow beyond the rainbow. He was said to see the future, particularly the future of the People. He was the last Chief to see in what they call the "Old Way". He tried to pass his way of seeing on to his son. But before he could do so, a great war broke out. The young son went to war and became a hero but returned broken hearted and bitter from defending a nation which needed him in war but despised him in peace. He turned further and further away from the Old Ways of the People. He refused the Curing Ceremony which could have healed his broken heart and instead found forgetfulness in drink.

He grew bitter against his father too, for his father had foreseen that he would not remain a hero in the White man's eyes. The son reasoned that his father's sight was useless if all he saw was disappointment without also seeing how to change those things that disappointed him. So, he never attempted to see in his father's way again.

The father's explanation for his son's alcoholism was that the youth had seen the horrors of battle without purpose and, as a

25

Figs. 2.1. THE SNAKE CLAN. Snake carvings are found throughout the Americas and are signatures of the Snake Clan of the Hopis. The figure on the following page, the Humpbacked Flute Player, is the symbol of the Flute Clan at St. Johns. Illustrations by Oswald White Bear Fredericks from The Book of the Hopi, *by Frank Waters. Copyright © 1963 by Frank Waters. All rights reserved. Reprinted by permission of Viking Penguin, a division of Penguin Books USA, Inc.*

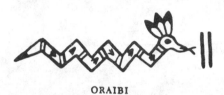

ORAIBI

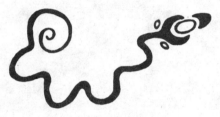

SERPENT MOUND

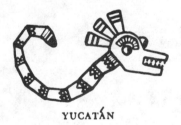

YUCATÁN

24 A Vision Quest, among the Native American Indians, is an essential part of a young man's (or, more rarely, a young woman's) initiation into adulthood. The youth is sent on a solitary vigil involving fasting and prayer in order to gain some sign of the presence and nature of his guardian spirit. Often the sign is a dream in which his guardian spirit appears to him, usually in animal form, instructs him and takes him on a visionary journey. Upon receiving these signs and visions the young warrior returns home, indicates his success and seeks out the shaman or medicine man for help in interpreting his vision.

result, never wanted to see again. He drank to keep the sight away.

Time passed and the Rainbow Chief began to have dreams of a young warrior to whom he could teach the Rainbow Way. But even though the Rainbow Chief continued to train other medicine apprentices, none of them ever saw the rainbow beyond the rainbow; nobody ever really understood what the Chief was talking about. Nevertheless, the People retained legends and stories about him, about the Medicine Chief who could see rainbows beyond rainbows, of one who knew the Rainbow Way so well he could look into a person's soul and know how it could be guided.

When the son was in his middle forties, still quite young and still an alcoholic, the Rainbow Chief went to be with the Sky People. Soon thereafter the son "found" God, became a born-again Christian, met and married a Christian lady and had a baby son. As that son grew into his late teens, he became discouraged with Christianity. A half-breed, he wanted to go back and find his father's way.

His search led him to Second Chance Mesa. There he discovered his tribe, met his people and found the apprentices that had worked with his grandfather. He decided to study with them, his own apprenticeship lasting eight years.

When it was time for his Vision Quest,24 one of his grandfather's apprentices, who had become the Tribal Medicine Chief, took the young man for a walk and asked, "Do you know who your grandfather was?"

"My father told me he was a crazy old man," replied the boy.

Upon hearing the boy's response, the Medicine Man proceeded to tell the story of

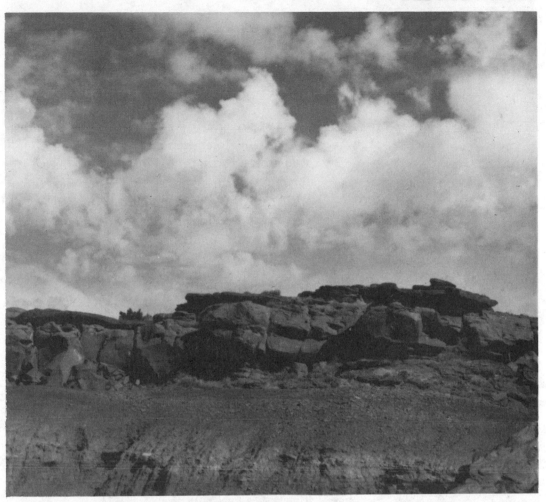

Fig. 2.2. *STORM OVER THE MESA.*
Photo by M.M. Smith/Techni-Visions.

the great Medicine Chief who had gone before him, the Chief who had seen the rainbows beyond rainbows.

Second Chance Mesa is a strange place given to extraordinary weather patterns, unusual light effect, and animals seen only by one person at a time. It was to this mysterious mesa that the Medicine Man sent the young warrior on his Vision Quest. The youth arrived at the mesa very early in the morning. For three days and two nights he fasted and prayed and waited for a vision.

On the afternoon of the third day a terrible storm came. Just before the storm began, a beautiful Eagle, who had been communicating with the young warrior all

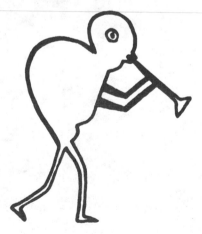

ST. JOHNS

27

day, flew in and screeched a warning to him as though to say, "By the way, this is it; this is the test." Then the Great Bird quickly disappeared.

The sun set, although the warrior never really saw it set because the sky was so dark. The storm kept up the entire night. It was all the young man could do to survive the torrent and the wind. The warrior was pelted with rain the whole night through. He was shivering, freezing, hungry. His body, having been in one position of prayer for nearly seventy-two hours, ached mercilessly. Still the young warrior sat and prayed. And waited. Sometime around sunrise, the storm ceased.

As dawn broke, the clouds began to separate. The whole mesa was bathed in light. It was a special quality of light, and the young warrior was not sure whether he was dreaming or whether he was awake. He looked across the valley floor. There he saw a Rainbow. He could see both ends of it as it arced across the valley. He looked upon it with the eyes and heart of a child, as though it were his first rainbow.

The warrior looked away, his eyes searching the sky for the Eagle. Within a moment the Great Bird appeared, swooped over him and screeched loudly. It proceeded to fly underneath the rainbow on the valley floor, and then up over it. That is when the young warrior noticed the second rainbow, above the first and separated by a golden layer. The Eagle continued its ascent and flew through yet another layer, revealing to the young warrior yet another rainbow. The Great Bird went still higher, through another golden layer, whereupon the warrior saw beyond that layer a fourth rainbow. Elated with his experience, he looked around at the shrubs on the mesa and realized he could see rainbows around the shrubs. A rabbit dashed by him and he could see a rainbow around the rabbit. In those few moments the young warrior realized that during the night he had gained his grandfather's Sight. Proudly he picked up his knife and went down the trail to find the Medicine Man. He found the teacher in his hut and told him what had happened. He told him about the Eagle screeching and about the terrible storm that seemed to come from nowhere. Finally the young warrior told the Medicine Man about the beautiful rainbows. "I can see a Rainbow around you now," he said, "Do you think that's what my grandfather saw?" The medicine teacher sat for a moment in silence. Then he looked at the warrior and said, "I don't know. No one has ever seen as your grandfather saw."

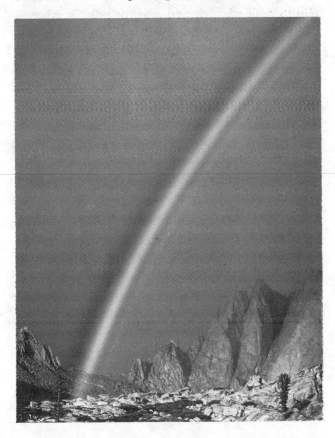

Fig. 2.3. RAINBOW OVER THE MESA. Photo by Robert E. Williams/Techni-Visions.

Wheels of Power

When a story like the one above is told in the Native American or Indian "Medicine World", it is told for a special purpose. These Medicine stories are obviously not about doctors or hospitals or aspirin, although they are intended to "heal" in some way. "Medicine" in this sense refers to the Sacred and the Spiritual. Medicine stories are similar, in a way, to the parables of Jesus in that the points they make are intended to connect the listeners to some sacred inner wisdom. Such a wisdom in the Indian world is called a Power. When one has a Power of any kind, it allows him to live more in harmony with the earth.

As we work or think in a Medicine Way, or as we pray in our hearts or hear a sacred story or parable and remember the context of the wisdom intended, we begin to reconnect parts of ourselves and to rediscover our own Powers. When we do this, we wait in silence as the young medicine warrior did for an internal message. We wait quietly to have that sacred wisdom or Power revealed. It is during such internal silence that we may begin to feel the chakra system, the subtle energies within.

This brings us to the primary issue at hand. Any discussion of chakras and auras must be undertaken by sanely and rationally answering the question: What do we know when we perceive them? In other words, what knowledge, what Power, what wisdom do we attain in the act of perceiving chakras and auras? Knowing that, how do we then utilize this Power for the betterment of mankind?

When the Rainbow Warrior first saw "the rainbow beyond the rainbow" he was elated, for he had achieved a level of awareness of spiritual significance. However, when he returned to the medicine chief who had agreed to supervise his Vision Quest, the young warrior discovered that his new awareness was beyond the experience and thus the comprehension of his supervisor. The folklore of most cultures distinguishes that which is living or life-giving from that which is not by referring to its "rainbow" or its "light". The medicine chief knew in his heart that rainbow patterns, or auras, exist around every living thing. But in spite of his sincere attempts to see the light, he could not. Consequently, as a mentor to the Rainbow Warrior, the medicine chief could only draw from a legendary, not an experiential knowledge of that light, of those rainbow patterns.

The Rainbow Warrior could have been contented with the personal joy he felt in his accomplishment. He could have stopped his process there. Instead, he chose to follow what he saw with a dedication to service and devotion to his grandfather's path. He chose to be an ever present servant to his tribe. Most significantly, he chose to examine the differences and understand the meaning in the Rainbow Patterns around every living thing. If each of us is to move beyond the legend to the reality, beyond the tradition to the experience of those Rainbow Patterns—of the chakra energies—we too must choose to look for them, to feel them around every living thing. Having once perceived them, we must then seek the meaning of these patterns. We must explore their historical roots but we must also follow the path of these energies into modern science.

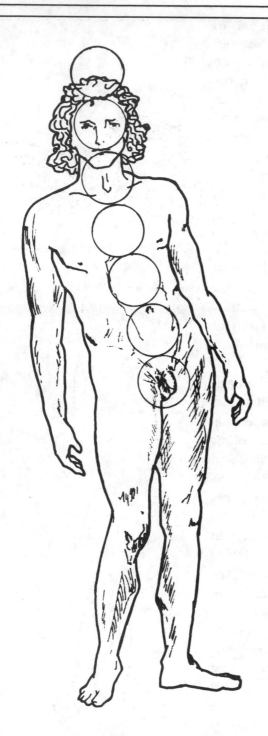

3 Color: Yellow

Seat of Mental Body
Adrenal (or Splenic) Center
Element: Air
Animal: Bird
Stone: Peridot, Topaz
Contains: Opinion
People: Friends, classmates,
　　　　intellectuals, politicians

2 Color: Orange

Seat of Emotional Body
Lymphatic Center
Element: Water
Animal: Fish
Stone: Aquamarine
Contains: Feeling
People: Those who teach us
　　　　feelings or to whom we
　　　　give feelings

1 Color: Red

Seat of Physical Body
Gonadic Center
Element: Fire
Animal: Snake
Stone: Ruby
Contains: Concept, original idea
People: Traditional (root)
　　　　relationships: Parents,
　　　　grandparents, etc.

*Fig. 2.4. CHAKRAS AND THEIR
TRADITIONAL COMPONENTS.*

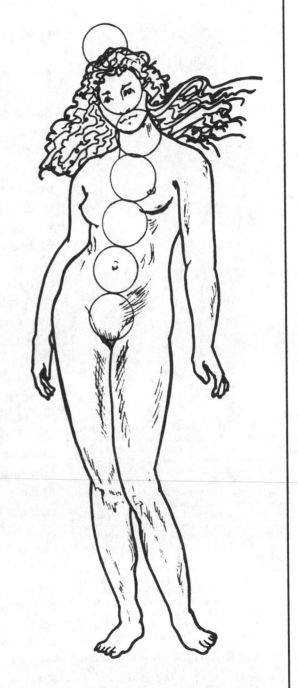

7 Color: White

Seat of Ketheric Body
Pituitary Center
Element: Magnetum
Animal: Kachina
Stone: Diamond
Contains: Release, surrender
People: Prophets, gurus, saints

6 Color: Violet

Seat of Celestial Body
Pineal Center
Element: Radium
Animal: All Spirits living or dead
Stone: Alexandrite
Contains: Inspiration/Insight
People: Spirit teachers,
   spiritual friends

5 Color: Blue

Seat of Etheric Body
Thyroid Center
Element: Ether
Animal: Human
Stone: Lapis or Sapphire
Contains: Expression
People: Religious leaders,
      divine rulers

4 Color: Green

Seat of Astral Body
Thymic Center
Element: Earth
Animal: Mammal (4-legged ally)
Stone: Emerald
Contains: Second feeling,
      (usually contrary to the first),
      transformation
People: "heart-chakra teachers"

Chakras and
Their Traditional Components

Wheels of Light

The word *chakra* is a Hindu word. The word literally means *"wheel of light"* in Sanskrit. While most traditions refer to seven major chakras,[25] some name fewer centers. Tibetan literature, for instance, identifies only six chakras.[26] It is generally understood, however, that when we refer to a chakra, we mean one of the seven major energy centers within the body. With the addition of the two higher chakras that exist outside the body—the *Atman* and the *Brahman*—there are actually nine chakras.

Each of the seven traditional chakras has a physical, an emotional, a creative and a celestial component. Besides these, each chakra has its own purpose or particular viewpoint based upon the area of consciousness which it influences. This area of consciousness is yet another component of the chakra. The ancient Yogis as well as the ancient Egyptians and Greeks called this component a *body*. This body is, again, simply an area or realm of existing or potential consciousness.

The specific body or purpose or *viewpoint* of each chakra dictates a particular attitude toward reality. Or, put another way, each chakra has a "Prime Directive". It has a purpose, a mind of its own; it is going somewhere. We could, for example, view all of life from a physical perspective—from our first chakra—if we so chose, as did, for instance, Rameses the Great, the renowned builder of Egypt and father of 144 children; he built

[25] The principle of the chakras first appears in the ancient Hindu *Upanishads* (the *Arunopnishad*, the *Yoga-shikka* and *Brihadaranyaka Upanishads*) of the Vedic texts. A later description of the chakras, their colors and powers can be found in the yoga text, *Gorakshashatakan*, written by the pundit Goraknath around the tenth century. Goraknath, commonly regarded as the founder of the Kahphata Yogis, who adhere to the discipline of Hatha Yoga, was considered a guru and living saint by the people of his day. For a summary of his chakra teachings, refer to Hiroshi Motoyama, *Theories of the Chakras: Bridge to Higher Consciousness*, Wheaton, Illinois: The Theosophical Publishing House, 1981. The *Yoga-shikka Upanishad* contains the most detailed passages concerning chakras. (See Chapter 1:168 and 1:172-175).

[26] See Rechung Rinpoche, *Tibetan Medicine*, Berkeley, California: University of California Press, 1976. See also W. Y. Evans-Wentz, *The Tibetan Book of the Dead*, New York: Oxford University Press, 1960.

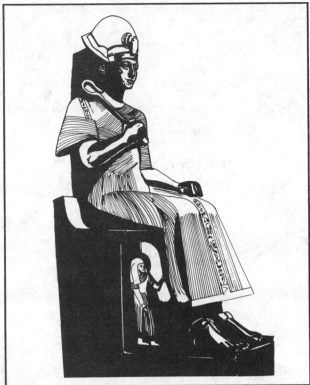

Fig. 2.5. *RAMESES THE GREAT*
Granite statue in Turin Museum, Italy.

great temples and statues, and his goal was to conquer the Hittites. He was very power-oriented and nothing stood in the way of his manifesting on a physical level. That is an example of a first chakra person. Many of the figures who have shaped the history of our planet might be considered first chakra people. Unfortunately, in our history books, many of the men and women whom we might term "first chakra oriented" have been (in)famous for their qualities of dominance, conquest, power, ambition and a driving need to express their vitality and prove their virility. These are qualities associated with the first chakra, whose viewpoint is to be and stay alive, no matter what the consequences. We will more completely examine the various components, qualities and particular viewpoint of each chakra in subsequent volumes.

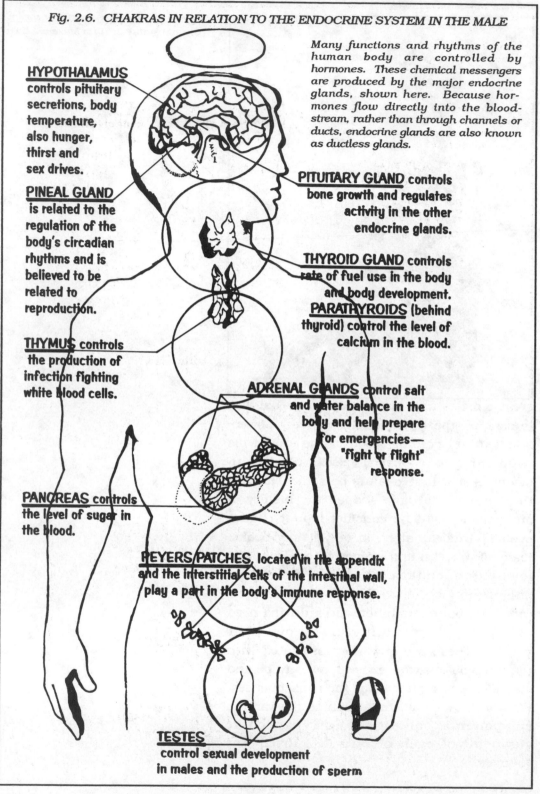

Fig. 2.6. *CHAKRAS IN RELATION TO THE ENDOCRINE SYSTEM IN THE MALE*

Many functions and rhythms of the human body are controlled by hormones. These chemical messengers are produced by the major endocrine glands, shown here. Because hormones flow directly into the bloodstream, rather than through channels or ducts, endocrine glands are also known as ductless glands.

HYPOTHALAMUS controls pituitary secretions, body temperature, also hunger, thirst and sex drives.

PINEAL GLAND is related to the regulation of the body's circadian rhythms and is believed to be related to reproduction.

THYMUS controls the production of infection fighting white blood cells.

PANCREAS controls the level of sugar in the blood.

PITUITARY GLAND controls bone growth and regulates activity in the other endocrine glands.

THYROID GLAND controls rate of fuel use in the body and body development. **PARATHYROIDS** (behind thyroid) control the level of calcium in the blood.

ADRENAL GLANDS control salt and water balance in the body and help prepare for emergencies— "fight or flight" response.

PEYERS PATCHES, located in the appendix and the interstitial cells of the intestinal wall, play a part in the body's immune response.

TESTES control sexual development in males and the production of sperm

Fig. 2.7. CHAKRAS IN RELATION TO THE ENDOCRINE SYSTEM IN THE FEMALE

In addition to the endocrine glands, several other organs also manu-facture hormones: the stomach, intestines, liver, kidneys and heart all contain groups of hormone-secreting cells. Hormone derives from the Greek word for "excite", but hormones can inhibit as well as stimulate bodily processes.

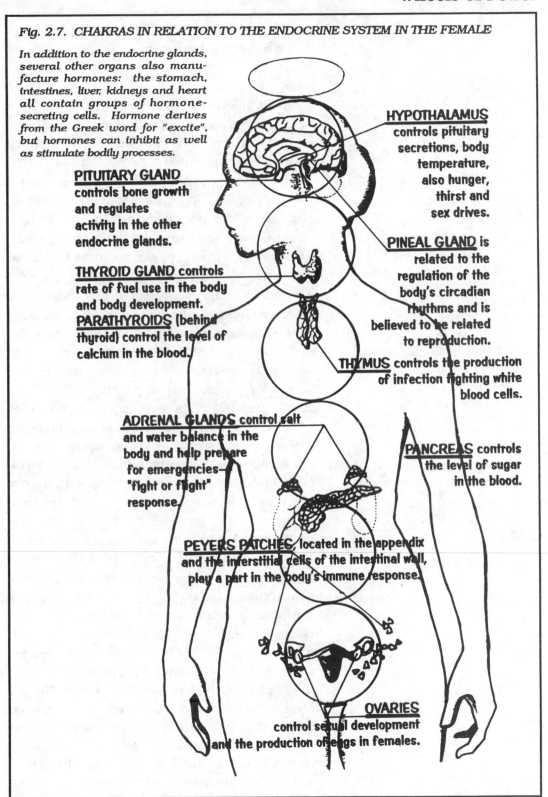

PITUITARY GLAND controls bone growth and regulates activity in the other endocrine glands.

THYROID GLAND controls rate of fuel use in the body and body development. **PARATHYROIDS** (behind thyroid) control the level of calcium in the blood.

ADRENAL GLANDS control salt and water balance in the body and help prepare for emergencies— "fight or flight" response.

HYPOTHALAMUS controls pituitary secretions, body temperature, also hunger, thirst and sex drives.

PINEAL GLAND is related to the regulation of the body's circadian rhythms and is believed to be related to reproduction.

THYMUS controls the production of infection fighting white blood cells.

PANCREAS controls the level of sugar in the blood.

PEYERS PATCHES, located in the appendix and the interstitial cells of the intestinal wall, play a part in the body's immune response.

OVARIES control sexual development and the production of eggs in females.

Secondary Chakras

Occasionally one of the ancient or modern mystical teachers will refer to a secondary chakra. In addition to the major chakras, there are 122 smaller secondary chakras throughout the body. Although this book's primary focus is on the seven major chakra centers, it is important to remember that both the primary and the secondary chakras have the same characteristics. To an aura reader, they appear as little cyclones; each is a whirling vortex of energy. Secondary chakras are smaller vortices than primary chakras. And while primary chakras are represented as being located along the spine (see Fig. 3.11), secondary chakras exist primarily wherever there is a joint in the body. Each place a bone touches a bone or a nerve plexus exists a secondary chakra is present. Consequently, secondary chakras are energy centers that are associated with a nerve plexus, a bone and a joint of some kind.

Though they are not major energy centers, these secondary chakras are important. The hips, for example, are important because they join the legs to the rest of the body. Much of our connective tissue (that tissue primarily responsible for carrying electromagnetic energy) is in our legs and buttocks, which represent around 38% of our body. Thus, if for any reason we are "cut off" at a level below the hips, 38% of the system that should be feeding the internal organs may not be giving us the vital energy, the life force—the Hindus call it prana—that we need to get through the day. Essentially, because of the way we think, we Americans create a pattern in our chakras and auras by which we "cut off" our legs from the rest of our body.

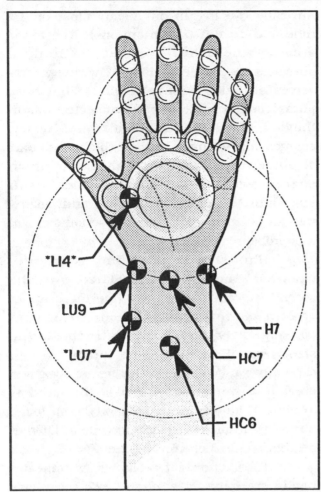

Fig. 2.8. CHAKRAS IN THE HANDS. The chakras in the hands are plentiful, and it is interesting how they relate to each other.. The meridian points are:

LI = Large Intestine
LU = Lung
H = Heart
HC is Heart Constrictor
    or Pericardium

Fig. 2.9. COLORS EMANATING FROM THE FINGERS. The energy emitting from each finger often corresponds to a specific color as indicated in the picture below. Computer drawings by M.M. Smith/Techni-Visions

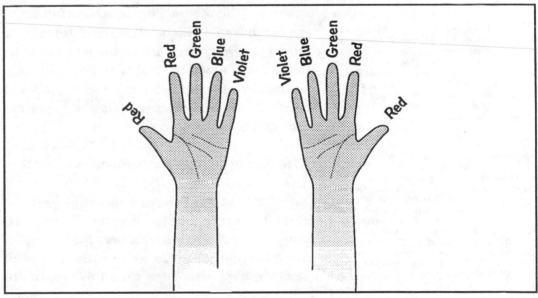

Aurically, we live in our heads most of the time and do not pay attention to the lower areas of the body. We tend to think of ourselves as intellectuals, and we view ourselves as being "above it all". That very phrase puts us into this disconnected way of thinking that is "a cut above". As a result, energetically we have "cut off" the bottom part of ourselves. When we realize how much energy and power, both physical and spiritual, is located in the legs and thighs, we can begin to recognize the seriousness of this problem.

Hands also contain secondary chakras. Hands are associated with the second trigram of the body (the three upper chakra centers) because our arms and consequently our hands attach to the shoulders. Hands are both functional and expressive; they express what we are doing and often how we think. Because the hand is "chakraful" (due to its many joints), each finger transmits a different color and thus a different frequency: red, blue, violet and green.[27]

Hips, shoulders, elbows, wrists and hands are only a few of the 122 secondary chakras. The relationship of some of these to major chakras will be discussed further in subsequent chapters and volumes. Let it be noted here, however, that a dysfunction of a secondary as well as a major chakra could detrimentally affect the efficiency of the entire chakra system.

The Seven Chakra Bodies [28]

The first chakra is the area of consciousness of the *physical body*; all physical sensation including, for example, pleasure and pain, as well as the powerful emotion, rage, emanates from this center. In

[27] Traditionally, both the thumb and forefinger channel red, the middle finger, green, the ring finger, blue, and the little finger, violet. However, this pattern varies according to the way one runs his or her own energy and how open one is energetically from the chest up. It may also be affected by physical problems such as, for example, a stiff neck.

[28] See the *Brihadaranyaka* and the *Yoga-shikka Upanishads*. Also refer to G.R.S. Mead, *Orpheus*, London, 1965 which explores the philosophy and rites of the Orphics (to which such Greeks as Pythagorus and Plato ascribed), and Edward Schure, *The Great Initiates*, trans. Gloria Rasberry, New York: Harper and Row, 1961. For a more recent discussion of "subtle bodies" refer to H. Motoyama, *Science and the Evolution of Consciousness*, Brookline, Massachusettes: Autumn Press, Inc., 1978, Chapter 5.

addition, all survival needs and self-preservation instincts are influenced by this body. The second chakra is the *emotional body* or realm; all emotions are processed here and under the dominion of this second center. The third center is the *mental* or *intellectual body* or realm; thoughts, opinions and judgments originate from this chakra and are controlled by it.

Whereas the lower three chakras—the physical, emotional and mental bodies—are self-evident and culturally more clearly understood, the upper chakras require more explanation. The fourth chakra, or the heart center, is identified as the *astral body* or plane; this is the first level beyond three-dimensional reality, that experiential level just above the physical, emotional, and intellectual planes. The astral is the realm or level of consciousness which bridges the dimensions of matter and spirit. It is believed to be the plane to which we travel in sleep. The astral level is the dream world. The astral plane also represents the level of consciousness wherein *transformation* and the *transpersonal* are made possible.

The fifth chakra is the *etheric body*. It is the first in the spiritual realm and as such it is the beginning of one's God-like abilities. The etheric body is, foremost, the template for the physical body. In other words, it is the perfect body, the "light body" which underlies our physical form. The etheric body is the spiritual underpinning or matrix for our physical being. It is a perfect hologram of our life or our life force. The etheric "substance" is thought to be the force that binds the universe together; therefore, if something *is*—physical, emotional, mental or spiritual —it has an etheric nature.[29] Because the etheric is the template for all physical reality,

29 Although of the spiritual realm, the etheric body has been described by some clairvoyants as a blue light or gauzy "web" that extends either around the outside of the physical body or exists within it, or both. One explanation for the phenomenon of "phantom limbs", or the experience of "physical sensation" in the area in which a severed limb previously existed, is that the etheric body, the undamaged template, is being experienced.

Fig. 2.10. THE SEVEN CHAKRA BODIES. See overleaf. Figures drawn by Charlotte Kaiser.

	COLOR	BODY	GLAND	ANIMAL
7	White	Ketheric	Pituitary	Kachina
6	Purple	Celestial	Pineal	Archetypes All Spirits living & dead
5	Blue	Etheric	Thyroid	Human & Hierophant
4	Green	Astral	Thymus	Mammal (4 legged)
3	Yellow	Mental	Adrenal (or Splenic)	Bird
2	Orange	Emotional	Peyer's Patches (or lymphatic)	Aquatic Animals
1	Red	Physical	Gonads	Snake

ELEMENT	GEMSTONE	CONTAINS	PEOPLE
Magnetum	Diamond	Release Surrender	Prophets Gurus Saints
Radium	Alexandrite	Inspiration Insight	Spirit teachers Spiritual friends
Ether	Lapis Sapphire	Expression	Religious leaders Divine rulers Pope, DaliLama Karmapa
Earth	Emerald	Second Feeling (usually contrary to first feeling)	Heart-chakra teachers Jesus, Yogananda Mother Teresa
Air	Topaz Peridot	Opinion	Friends Classmates intellectuals politicians
Water	Aquamarine	Feeling	Those who teach us feelings & to whom we give feelings Children, Spouses
Fire	Ruby	Concept Original Idea	Traditional root relationships: Parents Grandparents

the power of time, (especially in the sense of knowing the perfect time for doing something) and the power of speech and self-expression are also under the dominion of this body. Because the etheric is perfect, our concepts of justice, of truth and of perfection itself are all contained within this body or level of consciousness. The etheric body is like our perfect double; it represents our total and higher potential.[30]

The sixth chakra, often termed "the third eye", is the *celestial body,* and like the etheric, is of the spiritual realm. It is the world or body which holds our individual future and is also our access to that future. The term "celestial" derived from antiquity where it was believed that the future existed in space and that one day each of us would die and become a "star", thus returning to the divine celestial Light from which we had come. However, this would not occur until we had accumulated enough light (enlightenment) to illuminate a section of heaven.[31] The celestial body is that realm of light; and being associated with illumination, this body influences all that light enables us to "see". Put another way, the celestial body allows us to literally "see the light". It is the realm of "sight" in all of its various manifestations: clairvoyance, visualization, insight, foresight, inspiration, psychic phenomena and finally physical manifestation itself (from the thought, dream, fear, or other feeling to physical reality).

The seventh center, or the crown chakra, is the *ketheric body.* "Kether" in Hebrew simply means "crown".[32] The ketheric body controls and influences the area of consciousness known as the spirit or the *spiritual realm.* Within this body exists our spiritual life. The ketheric body is our place of mergence with God, the Oneness, the All.

[30] Manley P. Hall, Man: *Grand Symbol of the Mysteries,* Los Angeles: ©The Philosophical Research Society, Inc., 1972, pp .124-125.

[31] Manley P. Hall, *The Secret Teachings of All Ages,* Los Angeles: ©The Philosophical Research Society, Inc., 1977, p. XL. Also refer to Shure, op. cit. Chapter 33.

[32] H. P. Blavatasky, *Theosophical Glossary,* Los Angeles: The Theosophy Company, 1973, p. 177. The origin of the word is the *Kabbala,* the Jewish mystical tradition. Kether is the first of the ten Sefira.

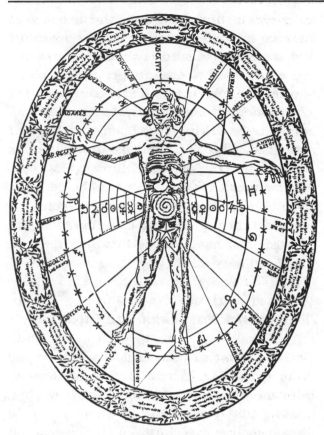

Fig. 2.11. THE BODY AS A MICRO-COSM. The border contains names of animal, mineral and vegetable substances. Their relationship to the corresponding parts of the body is shown by lines. The words on the lines indicate to which body part, organ or disease the herb or other substance is related. From Kircher's OEDIPUS AEGYPTIACUS.

The Body as a Microcosm

The concept of the human body as a symbolic representation of something greater is not a new idea. In Egyptian culture this idea can be traced back five or six thousand years to the most ancient extant Egyptian text.[33] The Chinese also have a system similar to that of the Egyptians.[34] Most of this symbology either sprouted from or existed side by side with the religion of that time. The basic tenet of every religion is that the soul is a spirit form or a life force that only temporarily lives in a body and that the body is merely its vehicle.

In modern thought, this concept appears as the microcosm/macrocosm theory, whereby everything in the outer world also exists in the inner world: the individual is a

[33]   Egyptian *Book of the Dead* (which the Egyptians called the book of the *Coming Forth* (from death) *By Day*). These are actually some 2,000 papyrus rolls, dating from the Pyramids (some before), found in various tombs and distinguished by formulas to guide the dead. (G. Maspero, *The Dawn of Civilization: Egypt and Chaldea*, London: 1897, p. 102-03. Cited by Will Durant, *The Story of Civilization I: Our Oriental Heritage*, New York: Simon and Schuster, 1954, p. 203).

[34]   Taoism, as revealed in its physical discipline and meditation process, views the body and spirit in much the same way as the ancient Egyptians. There is evidence that communication existed between the Egyptians, Tibetans and Chinese as early as 800 BC (refer to James A. Hurtak, "The Human System: An Open-Ended Universe" in *Energies of Consciousness*, op. cit.)

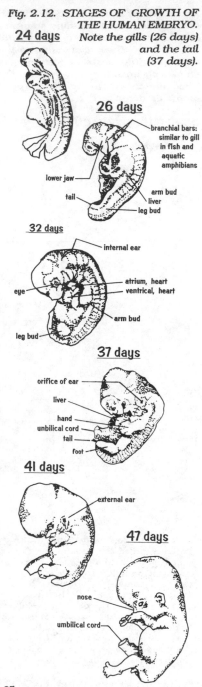

Fig. 2.12. STAGES OF GROWTH OF THE HUMAN EMBRYO.
Note the gills (26 days) and the tail (37 days).

24 days

26 days

branchial bars: similar to gill in fish and aquatic amphibians

lower jaw

tail

arm bud
liver
leg bud

32 days

internal ear

eye

atrium, heart
ventrical, heart

arm bud

leg bud

37 days

orifice of ear

liver

hand
unbilical cord
tail
foot

41 days

external ear

47 days

nose

umbilical cord

35 This idea can be traced from the ancient philosophies of the Hindus, Egyptians, Greeks and Romans to those of the Kabbalists, alchemists and Freemasons and into modern science. Cf. Hall, *Man,* op. cit. Chapter III and Hall, *The Secret Teachings of All Ages,* op. cit. pp. LXXIII - LXXVI.

microcosm of humanity; the atom is a microcosm of the universe.[35] The idea that the inner world and the outer world are representations of one another suggests that if the ancient idea of chakras and the corresponding bodies (physical, emotional, mental, astral, and so on), is closely examined, a specific relationship between the chakras and the organs of the physical body can be found. In the following chapters and volumes we will explore the ways in which the organs reflect shifts in the energy of the chakras, especially those to which they are related in frequency.

Animal and Elemental Nature of the Chakras

Ontogeny recapitulates phylogeny. This scientific theory which most of us remember from high school biology class means that the evolution of a species is repeated in the evolution of the individual. Thus, as embryos, each of us passed through all of the stages of growth in nine months which corresponded to man's three billion year evolution from a single-celled to a multi-celled organism. Theoretically, as man moves toward mergence with God, he is more evolved than the lower stages of creation. However, it is a scientific observation that the human fetus in utero goes through first a serpent stage, then a fish stage where it has gills before it begins to develop lungs and take on higher life form. This evolutionary cycle is reflected in metaphysical doctrine.

Fifteen thousand years ago this cycle was known to the American Indians and symbolized by them in the chakra system. (A similar symbology was developed by the

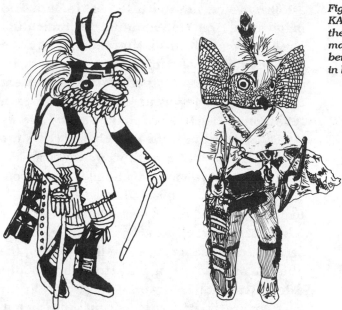

Egyptians nearly 50,000 years ago.[36]) Traditionally, according to American Indian lore, the lower chakras are aligned to animal forms. The first chakra is the snake, the second chakra is fish, the third chakra is bird or fowl, the fourth is mammal, and man resides in the fifth center. The sixth chakra takes man one step further into the collective and the spiritual, since again, according to Native American tradition, it is aligned with *all* spirits, living and dead. Finally, the seventh chakra is the *Kachina*, the living symbol of the Universal Spirit which embodies all animate matter.

It was the Egyptian priest-scribe, Tehuty, more familiarly known in myth and legend by his Greek name, Hermes,[37] who is first credited with defining the elementary nature of the chakra system some 50,000 years ago.

According to Hermetic tradition,[38] as we progress up the chakras from the first to the seventh, the associative elements in order

[36] Oral tradition, Egyptian priesthood. Much of Arab legend also traces Egyptian history back many thousands of years. In his book, *Secrets of the Great Pyramid* (New York: Harper & Row, 1971), Peter Tompkins cites an Arab historian, Abu Zeyd el Balkhy, who quotes an ancient inscription referring to the building of the Great Pyramid as having taken place when the "Lyre was in the Constellation of Cancer". An interpretation of this places the date of the construction of the Great Pyramid at around 71,000 years before Christ.

[37] Volume Four contains a more complete discussion of Tehuty-Hermes-Thoth and Hermetism.

[38] *Hermetica*, ed. and trans. from the Greek and Latin by Walter Scott, in four volumes, Oxford: Clarendon Press, 1924 - 1936.

Fig. 2.14. *TEHUTY-THOTH, THE IBIS-HEADED. From a bas-relief limestone. Abydos, Temple of Seti, XIXth Dynasty.*

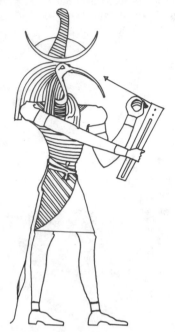

Fig. 2.15. *A GREEK FORM OF HERMES, THE DOG-HEADED. From Bryant's Mythology.*

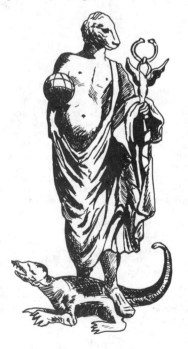

are fire, water, air, earth, ether, radium and magnetum. As we examine the individual chakras we will find that each chakra's particular viewpoint of life grows out of its elemental nature. In other words, the element that each center represents becomes a reflection of what that chakra views life as being. For instance, the first chakra views fire as life. The second chakra views water as life. The third chakra views air as life, and so on. Each chakra has a viewpoint that it maintains, based on its elemental nature.

This particular separation of elements serves a purpose as we move into viewing the chakra system as a way to process our external and internal worlds. The *fire* in the first chakra sparks *the concept* into being. The elements which follow play a role in the step-by-step destiny of that concept. *Water* comes after fire, because if we skip our feeling about that concept, as the fire combines with *air* (thought or opinion), oxygen (judgment or opinion) will mix with that flame and it will flare. Water is in the second chakra in case we need to put out that spark before it gets out of control. If we fail in this, once oxygen has been added and the flame grows larger, we again have an opportunity to smother it with *earth* (a second feeling). This process is available to us should we fail to move the concept though the chakra system *without* being able to *transmute* it at each stage into its next appropriate form—from a physical awareness of the concept to a feeling about it, to a thought or opinion about it and on to a second feeling about it. The heart chakra allows us this second feeling about the initial concept. It is that second feeling which then lets us decide whether or not the concept should be spoken. This transmutation of data at each chakra is a more appropriate transformation process: the original spark which has grown to a flame may now be transmuted into *ether, radium* and *magnetum* [39] respectively. The flame, then, becomes gas and finally energy itself, where it began. The particular nature of the chakra elements thus makes it possible to either stop the concept, the flow of energy, at any chakra or else, when used most efficiently, the individual chakra elements become the mechanism by which each chakra is able to transmute data so as to permit us to process our external and internal worlds completely.

Religious Perspectives of the Chakras

The major religions of the world all emphasize a different chakra or combination of chakras. These emphases are apparent in such things as prayer practice, ritual and the stated values of a particular group. The emphasis of Judaism, for example, is highly intellectual or third chakra, while the Islamic prayer posture of forehead, or sixth chakra, to the ground demonstrates an entirely different focus. Christianity's stated emphasis is love, specifically the love and "heart" of Jesus.

Ultimately, the entire development of a culture may center around a particular area of consciousness, often called "Deity" or "God" or "the One True Path". It is as though religious leaders view a group of people, consider their strengths and deficiencies and decide that a certain chakra or its associative values is what is needed by the group because these values are absent from the culture. We do not need God for what we have; we need God for what we lack. The way in which we are not like God is that toward which we seek to evolve.

[39] As yet *magnetum*, which contains properties of magnetism among other things, is unknown to modern science. However, this element is noted in the *Hermetica* and was probably known to ancient and medieval alchemists.

Fig. 2.16. THE VIRGIN BIRTH. The goddess Nut (The Sky) swallows and gives birth to the Sun. A.D. 1st-4th century. From painted ceiling relief, Temple of Hathor, Denderah, Egypt.

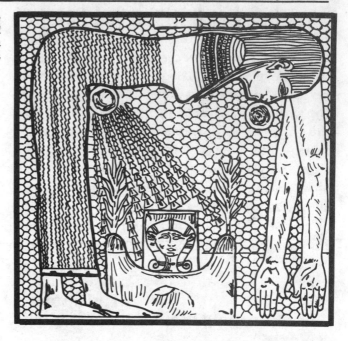

Clearly we will probably never know whether the process was so intentional, since most of the so called words of the founders of religions are apocryphal. What we do know is that:

> All powerful initiators have perceived in one moment of their lives the radiance of central truth, but the light which they drew from it was refracted and colored according to their genius, their mission, their particular time and place.[40]

Historical Perspectives

History of Chakras in the West: Theosophists' Theory

Historically the idea of chakra energies can be found in the West within the rituals of the ancient Greek mystery schools of Eleusis

[40]   Shure, op. cit., p. 169.

and Delphi as well as among the practices of early Christian mystics and Hermetics. The whole idea of chakras comes into Western mysticism again around the turn of the century. The early British Theosophists, Alice Bailey's group and the arcane school, traveled to India, "became enlightened", returned and wrote about chakras. In addition, the Rev. Charles Leadbeater and Annie Besant contributed their own literature on the chakras.[41] These Theosophists made certain assumptions from what they learned about chakras and what they knew about spirituality. Those assumptions may or may not be accurate.

They thought that higher *vibrations* or *frequencies* were limited to the upper chakras and lower *vibrations* to the lower chakras. What this idea did was to "split" the body in half, so that the lower energies were the "bad energies" and the upper energies were the "good" ones. It is not surprising to find a group of upper-class Victorian British gentry deciding that emotionalism was bad. They were validating a position they already held and visited India collecting data to support their belief. Interestingly, nothing in Hindu lore teaches that emotionalism is bad. What is bad is the misuse of emotionalism and the resulting sickness and imbalance this creates in life.

The Two Worlds of the Chakras

Although in ancient sources the chakras are not separated into "bad" chakras and "good" chakras, there is a basic distinction between the lower centers and the upper centers. They each represent a different three-dimensional world. The three-dimensional world of the lower chakras (the

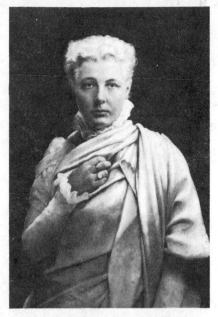

Fig. 2.17. Photo of ANNIE BESANT AND REV. CHARLES LEADBEATER courtesy of the Theosophical Publishing House, Wheaton, IL.

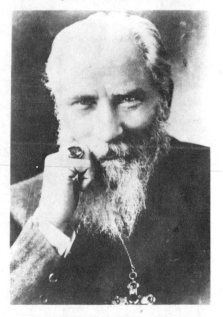

[41] Annie Besant and C.W. Leadbeater, *The Inner Life*, Wheaton, Illinois: The Theosophical Publishing House, 1978, and C.W. Leadbeater, *The Chakras*, Madras, India: The Theosophical Publishing House, 1927 (Available from Quest Books, Wheaton, Illinois)

first, second and third) is mankind's world, and the three-dimensional world of the upper chakras (the fifth, sixth and seventh) is God's world. (The fourth chakra acts as the transition between these two worlds.) In fact, it will become more evident as each chakra is individually investigated that there exists within each of us a continuous battle between the needs of our lower chakras and the expectations of our higher ones. This does not mean, however, the lower chakras are "bad" and the upper chakras are "good". As the chakras and their symbology are examined, it is my hope that this idea can finally be put to rest. In reality, the lowest chakra, the first, has some very high frequency—still within the same color band (red) but of a higher frequency—that is very powerful and useful. It is the lower frequencies we are trying to break with, not the lower chakras.

Chapter Three

WHAT IS AN AURA?

Auric Field: Field of Life

The first modern description of chakra energies or of what we call the aura or auric field was made by Sir Isaac Newton in 1729 in his second paper on light and colors. In this paper Newton spoke of an "electromagnetic" light, a "subtle, vibrating, electric and elastic medium" that was excitable AND exhibited phenomena such as repulsion, attraction, sensation and motion, anticipating in many ways the electromagnetic field theories of Michael Faraday and James Clerk Maxwell a hundred years later.[42]

It was not until this century, however, that the body's electrical nature became a fact of science. Beginning in the early 1930's Dr. Harold Saxton Burr spent over forty years scientifically researching what he called electro-dynamic or "L-fields" (the "L" stands for "Life"). These L-fields were detected and measured in men and women, in animals, trees, plants, seeds, eggs and even in one of the lowest life forms, slime-molds.[43] Burr theorizes that the L-field is responsible for the body's capacity to regenerate new cells which act and function precisely as did the cells which they have replaced. The analogy he uses is that of a jelly mold. "When a cook looks at a jelly mold, she knows the shape of the jelly she will turn out of it." In the same

[42] John Pierrakos, "The Human Energy Field" in *The Energies of Consciousness*, op. cit.. Michael Faraday (1791-1867) was a British physicist and chemist who discovered the phenomenon of electromagnetic induction—the production of electric current by a change in magnetic intensity—as well as the rotation of the plane of polarization (plane of vibration) of a light beam by a magnetic field (See Faraday effect). James Clerk Maxwell (1831-1879) was a Scottish physicist whose fame rests upon his formulation of electromagnetic theory itself (See Maxwell's equations). Maxwell has been ranked with Newton for the fundamental nature of his contributions to science. Newton's original description of the "electromagnetic" light can be found in his *Mathematical Principles of Natural Philosophy*, Berkeley, California: University of California Press, 1934 (originally printed in 1729).

[43] Burr, op. cit., p. 6.

way, "the electro-dynamic field of the body serves as a matrix or mold, which preserves the 'shape' or arrangement of any material poured into it, however often the material may be changed." Furthermore, this "invisible" and "intangible" field "can reveal the future 'shape' or arrangement of the materials it will mold."[44] In other words, an abnormality in the electro-dynamic field can "give warning of something 'out-of-shape' in the body, sometimes in advance of actual symptoms."[45] A healer can detect these electro-dynamic or energy inconsistencies through touch or sight; certainly, they may be detected instrumentally (through biofeedback mechanisms, for example).[46] With such forewarning, preventative action, whether a specific medical or psychological process or a rebalancing of energies through healing, may then be taken.

Over the past twenty years, the research of New York orthopedic surgeon Robert O. Becker and his colleagues has established with certainty the relationship between regeneration and electrical currents in living things. The flow of electrons (electric current) moving through the perineural cells[47] of the nervous system and the resultant magnetic field are the factors which affect an organism's ability to sense and evaluate damage occurring anywhere in the body; this electromagnetic flow also provides cells with the appropriate electrical environment to either sustain health within an uninjured cell or stimulate healing in a damaged cell.[48] This same perineural structure is the passageway utilized by healers when they channel energy into a client to bring about healing.[49] Both the L-field of Burr and the regeneration research of Becker have shed scientific light on the

---

[44] Ibid., p. 5.

[45] Ibid., p. 6.

[46] Biofeedback is a technique of self-training utilizing the aid of electronic devices. The purpose of this self-training is the control and modification of involuntary physical functions, such as blood pressure or heartbeat, and often that of certain emotional states, such as anxiety or depression.

[47] Perineural cells are cells containing bundles of nerve fibres surrounded by an extensive layer of connective tissue.

[48] See Becker and Selden, op. cit., Chapter 13.

[49] Cf. note 67 Chapter Four.

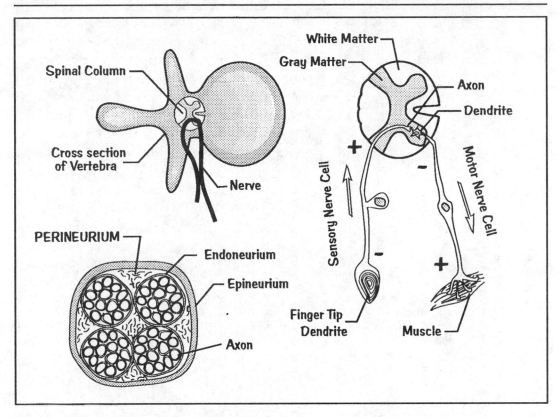

electromagnetic nature of the human body and consequently on the underlying electromagnetic nature of the chakra energies of the auric field.

The auric field is a metaphor for life. In other words, a person's energy field or the individual aura around the body, which is created and controlled by the chakras, reflects how one's life actually is lived; it mirrors the flow of that life. In this way, the auric field becomes more than a symbol for life: The aura is life.

Fig. 3.1. FLOW OF ENERGY THROUGH THE PERINEURAL CELLS. A cross section of the nerve bundles is shown in the lower left hand corner of the figure. Computer drawing by M.M. Smith/Techni-Visions.

Vibration, Color and Harmonics of the Aura

Our *auric* or *electromagnetic field* is generated by the spinning of the chakras. As it spins, each chakra produces its own electromagnetic field. This field then

Fig. 3.2. ELECTROMAGNETIC RADIATION. See Overleaf.

ELECTROMAGNETIC RADIATION and ITS SPECTRUM

Electromagnetic radiation is the propagation of energy through space by means of electric and magnetic fields that vary in time. This radiation may be characterized in accordance with the wave theory, either by its wavelength or by its frequency. **Frequency** is the number of waves passing a certain point in one second, shown in Figure 3.4. **Wave length** is the length of one full wave, or the distance travelled (at the speed of light) in one oscillation. Mathematically these two terms are inversely related to each other by the formula, frequency = propagation-velocity/wave length. The orderly arrangement of radiation according to wavelength or frequency is called the **electromagnetic spectrum.**

Although radiation is the more common term, electromagnetism can also be thought of as a field. The field exists in space around an object. It has two parts: the electric field and the magnetic field. The magnetic field can be measured by forces acting on certain kinds of materials such as iron. The electric field can be measured by forces acting on electrically charged particles. These two fields always coexist with the same intensity at a given location and instant in time. Hence, they are really parts of the same field, hence electromagnetic. Any body containing electric current (which can be macro or microscopic) possesses an electromagnetic field. If the field is static (does not vary with time), it does not transmit energy. In the special case where the field is dynamic (which is caused by varying or oscillating current in a body), variation in field intensity appears as waves radiating outwards from the source body. These waves transmit energy and are called electromagnetic radiation. Objects with an electrical current exhibit a comparable electromagnetic field. The waves behave as streams of massless, chargeless particles called photons

and include an electric field and a magnetic field perpendicular to the wave and to each other as illustrated in Fig. 3.4. Static fields are often called potential because their energy is in storage. Dynamic fields are so called because their intensity varies with time; these fields are referred to as kinetic, since motion is a part of their description. For further description of potential and kinetic, see Figure 3.8.

Electromagnetic radiation includes an enormous range of frequencies as the chart below depicts. The only energy we can see visually exists in a very narrow band width indicated on the chart. Above that, the higher ultraviolet, x-rays and gamma rays are called ionizing because of their ability to create highly reactive ions where they don't belong, as with nuclear radiation. Below visible light the waves are non-ionizing. Infrared waves are felt as heat, while microwave and radio frequencies are used for communication. This portion of the spectrum is arbitrarily broken up into frequencies with initials we all have heard—extremely high (EHF), superhigh (SHF), ultrahigh (UHF), very high (VHF), high (HF), medium (MF), low (LF), very low (VL) and extremely low frequencies (ELF). Brain waves are the lowest on the spectrum varying from .5 to 35 cycles per second. Special instrumentation (or second sight) is required to detect or see these lower frequency waves. . . . or any frequencies other than the tiny band of frequency allotted to visible light.

_____

Excerpted from the Encyclopaedia Britannica, Vol. 18, 1985 and Becker, The Body Electric, op. cit..

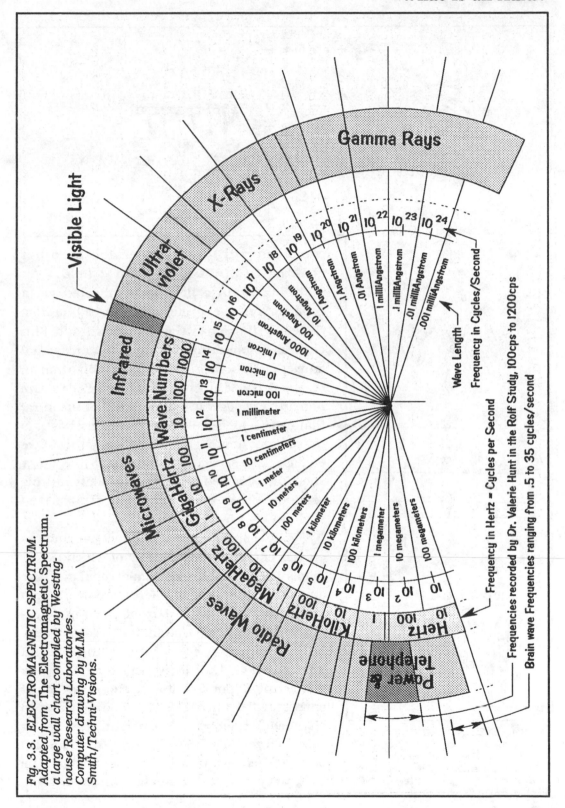

Fig. 3.3. *ELECTROMAGNETIC SPECTRUM.*
Adapted from The Electromagnetic Spectrum, a large wall chart compiled by Westing-house Research Laboratories. Computer drawing by M.M. Smith/Techni-Visions.

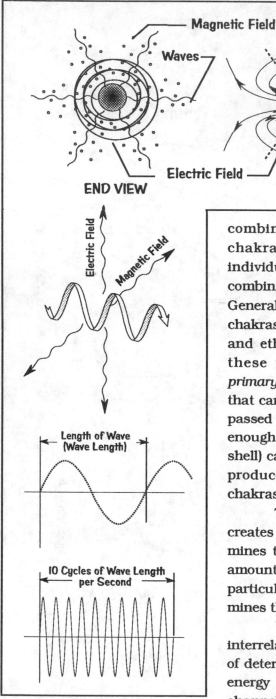

END VIEW

SIDE VIEW

Magnetic Field

Waves

Waves

Electric Field

Electric Field

Magnetic Field

Length of Wave
(Wave Length)

10 Cycles of Wave Length
per Second

Fig. 3.4. ELECTROMAGNETIC WAVE. Definitions of wave length, frequency and the direction of the magnetic and electric fields emitting from an electro-magnetic wave. Computer drawing by M.M. Smith/Techni-Visions.

combines with fields generated by other chakras to produce the auric field. An individual's auric field is manifested via a combination of energies from three chakras. Generally these are the first, third and fifth chakras empowering the physical, intellectual and etheric bodies. It is a combination of these three chakras that produces the *primary auric field* (the inner shell of the aura) that can be physically felt by the hand as it is passed over another's body. If one is sensitive enough, the *secondary auric field* (the outer shell) can also be felt. This secondary aura is produced from the interaction of all seven chakras.

The spinning of the individual chakras creates energy, the frequency of which determines the color of a particular chakra. The amount or intensity of energy produced by a particular chakra or group of chakras determines the color that dominates the auric field.

Vibration, color and *sound* are all interrelated and all three represent a means of determining or monitoring the *frequency* of energy in the auric field. When a healer is channeling energy into a person, the healer will often feel a vibration within the muscles of his or her own body. Correspondingly, the client may also feel a similar vibration. This vibration is directly related to the color of energy being channeled. Thus, the healer can kinesthetically sense (and thereby know without "seeing") the color of energy being channeled into a client. Some healers are able to hear (clairaudiently) the sound of the color being channeled. In this way they are able to monitor and know what color energy they are transferring into the client. In addition to "feeling" and "hearing" color,

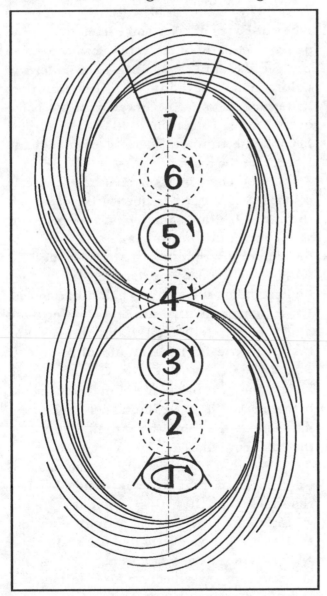

Fig. 3.5. THE CREATION OF THE PRIMARY AURIC FIELD. A combination of energies from chakras one, three and five generates the inner shell of the aura. Computer drawing by M.M. Smith/Techni-Visions.

clairvoyants are able to see energies and auric fields.[50] As a point of clarification, when reference is made to the color of energy, not only the visible light spectrum is intended but also the non-visible frequency bands as well; x-rays, gamma rays, ultraviolet, infra-red, and microwave bands are included in this category. When clairvoyants see the auric field, they may be "reading" one or more of these frequency bands (see Fig. 3.3).

The auric field actually exists in different layers of color sometimes referred to as *harmonics*. In other words, for people who can see the aura, it appears as a pattern of colors near the body and then another pattern of colors farther away from the body, and so on. This is just like the rainbow beyond the rainbow seen by the Medicine Warrior on the mesa.

The color in each chakra likewise is composed of varying frequency bands within the range of that same color. Since color, vibration and sound are all ways of determining frequency, perhaps a musical analogy will be of assistance in further understanding the idea of chakra harmonics. Those frequencies that are an octave or more apart may be termed harmonics. For instance, the first harmonic of middle C would be C above middle C, one octave higher; the next harmonic of middle C would be the next fifth above the higher C; the next harmonic is the third above that, followed by the fifth above that, and so on.

When a note is struck on the piano, a wave form of that note is emitted. The resonance of that first wave excites a vibration in other notes of mathematical equivalence. If we slowly depress and hold a piano key so it does not sound, then strike and release a key an octave lower, a tone will

[50] It is believed that those who have the ability to see auric color do so by "speeding up" the normal process of visual perception.

60

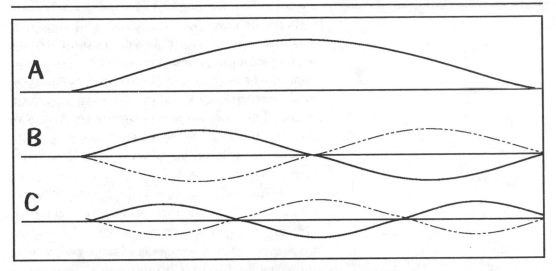

be heard in the depressed key. The depressed note is the first harmonic of the lower, or *fundamental* note. The second note vibrates because its natural frequency (measured in cycles per second) is triggered into movement by a complementary frequency in the original note. This phenomenon is known as *harmonic*, or *sympathetic vibration*. Each harmonic is a mathematical multiple (in cycles per second) of the fundamental note.

The research conducted by Dr. Valerie Hunt at UCLA did, in fact, match sound to color; vibration and color correlated directly. Furthermore, our equipment was able to measure seven (and there may be more) harmonics or varying frequency bands of (sound, vibration and) color of each chakra.[51]

The frequencies of visible color have a harmonic relationship to the frequencies of auric color; auric colors may exist in both lower and higher harmonics of visible color.[52] Let us use the example of a woman wearing a red blouse. That red blouse reflects the visible light color red; red here simply indicates a hue or pigment. If we see red in the *aura* of the woman, however, that red could indicate either pain or anger. These two

Fig. 3.6. MUSICAL HARMONIC OF A VIBRATING STRING.
A. Vibration of an open string. This is the fundamental frequency of the string.
B. If the string is stopped to form two equal lengths, each being half of the original, then the frequency doubles, thereby producing the first harmonic.
C. If the string is stopped to form three equal lengths, each being one third of the original, then the frequency doubles again, thereby producing the second harmonic.

51   Hunt, op. cit. Refer to Appendix for discussion and illustration of the frequency analysis of the chakras or auric colors.

52   Although this was not among the findings of the Rolf Study, more recent research into energy field phenomenon performed by Dr. Hunt has provided some exciting new findings regarding the auric field and corresponding frequencies and harmonics. This research will soon be available in Dr. Hunt's forthcoming book.

reds in the aura look identical, but they are not the same. The lower two or three harmonics of the color red reflect pain in the physical body. In the higher red harmonics (or vibrations) there exists the same drive or action that pain excites someone to, but it is not pain itself. At least it is not physical pain; it could be existential pain. It could also be rage or anger.

As the frequency or harmonics or vibration of energy our body channels gets slower we become more physical; as the frequency of this energy gets faster we become more esoteric, less physical. There is a definite continuum from low to high frequency, and in the esoteric world we are trying to channel and maintain finer and higher frequencies (vibrations).

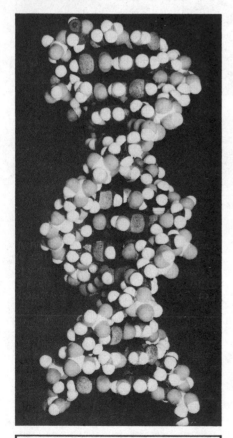

Fig. 3.7. DNA MOLECULE. Ball and Stick Model. Note how the DNA spiral corresponds to the flow of energy up the chakra system. Omicron/Photo Researchers, Inc.

Fig. 3.8. ENERGY AND MATTER. A scientific perspective. See overleaf.

Energy: The Basic Component of the Body

The only thing that affects our body is the level and kind of energy to which it is exposed. If we view the body as energy and consider everything that affects the body according to an energy model, we begin to understand the relationship between chemicals and the body, food and the body, light and the body, sound and the body, and the relationship between ourselves and others. Using this model, we come to see the body as more than a simple internal combustion engine that works only on food and water. We arrive at a more subtle understanding of the electrochemical, energy production (or reduction) value of not only our food intake but of anything we ingest. We are no less affected by air pollution, noise pollution or "people pollution": if we are

•••••••••••••**AS SCIENCE SEES IT**••••••••••••••

The Encyclopaedia Britannica states that the question "What is energy . . . or matter?" correctly belongs in the realm of metaphysics, whereas the understanding of how these subjects relate to the universe and other physical phenomena belongs to physics. Recently the two disciplines have come much closer together as a more thorough understanding of the nature of energies and the universe emerges.

ENERGY

Technically speaking, **energy** is most simply defined as the capacity for doing work. It appears in many forms—gravitational, heat, chemical, kinetic, elastic, electrical, radiant, nuclear, mass energy—and may be converted from one form to another. No matter what the medium, it can always be expressed by the equivalent work done. The work done is defined as the amount of force (F) multiplied by the distance (s) through which the force acts. Energy is most often associated with a material body; however, it can also be independent of matter as with light and other wave forms from the electromagnetic spectrum.

The Law of Conservation of Energy states that the total amount of energy in the universe remains constant. In other words, energy can be transformed but it cannot be created or destroyed. At any time energy and the capacity for doing work is said to exist, it is in one of two forms—kinetic or potential. Potential energy is energy in storage which exists by reason of a body's position in a force field, while kinetic energy exists by reason of a body's motion. An example of the interaction of these two energies is a ball thrown upward. At a certain point, the ball stops, turns around and returns to earth. At its highest point, it is said to have potential energy which will be returned in the form of kinetic energy as it falls back to earth and its starting point. Electric potential occurs in an electric field and is defined as the the amount of work required to move a positive charge through the field from infinity to a defined point.

Power is a term often associated with energy. Its definition is simply the time rate at which energy or work (F * s) is transformed from one form of energy to another. For example, an engine has power because it transforms chemical energy into mechanical energy.

When particles of the atom interact mechanically, such as to form ions, or energy radiates in the form of an electromagnetic wave, transfers of energy can occur. Electric and magnetic fields are intimately a part of the absorption or emission that permits the transfer of energy.

MATTER

Matter is distinguished from energy because it occupies space and has mass—it weighs something. Matter is made up of atoms, which consist of very small particles. The nucleus, or center part of the atom, contains positively charged protons and neutrons. Neutrons have no charge at all and are about the same mass as .the proton. Tiny, negatively charged particles, called electrons, revolve about the nucleus, in the same manner as the planets revolve about the sun. Protons are about 1800 times more massive than the electron. The diameter of the electron is 0.00000000000022 inches—very small indeed. It is the speed (186,000 miles/second), not the tiny size, that makes them capable of generating large amounts of energy. The number of protons, electrons and neutrons determines the resulting **element** (see Fig 3.9). Elements combine to create molecules which build a **substance** (one kind) or a **compound** (two or more elements). Organic chemistry is the study of compounds containing the substance carbon. Our bodies and the food we eat contain a huge variety of carbon, hydrogen and oxygen atoms combined to create many different molecular compounds.

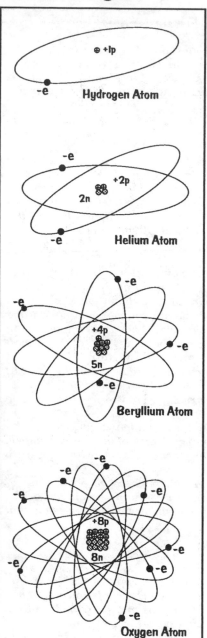

Hydrogen Atom

Helium Atom

Beryllium Atom

Oxygen Atom

When elements combine to form a compound, a transfer of electrons occurs. For example, when sodium and chlorine combine to form sodium chloride, or salt, each molecule consists of one sodium atom and one chlorine atom. The bond is formed by the transfer of **one** electron from the sodium atom to the mating chlorine atom. Because the electron has a negative (-) charge, the sodium atom is left with a positive (+) charge and the chlorine atom becomes positive. Since opposite charges attract, the atoms are tightly and stably bonded together.

Under certain conditions this stable bond can be broken but doing so is usually difficult and may require substantial energy input into the process—as in the extraction of metals from ore. With certain compounds, the molecular bond can be broken by being **dissolved** in water to form a **solution**. Sodium chloride dissolved in water causes the sodium and chlorine atoms to temporarily become disassociated. The individual atoms, which retain their positive or negative electrical charges while wandering individually through the solution, are called ions. Chemically pure water cannot transmit an electrical current because it contains no ions. An aqueous salt solution, however, can transmit current through the migration of electrically charged ions.

Water occurring in natural bodies, particularly oceans, is highly ionized with various dissolved minerals. The ions create the environment where electricity conducts easily. . . . and healing can occur.

For more complete explanations, see the Encyclopaedia Britannica, 15th Ed., Vol.18, 1985.

Fig. 3.9. ATOMS. AND IONS. A variety of atoms with their appropriate particles are shown. Below, the sodium and chlorine atoms become sodium and chloride ions. The single electron in the sodium outer shell readily transfers to the chlorine, which has a "gap" in its outer shell. Mobility of these electrically charged ions is the means for electrical conduction. Computer drawings by M.M. Smith/Techni-Visions.

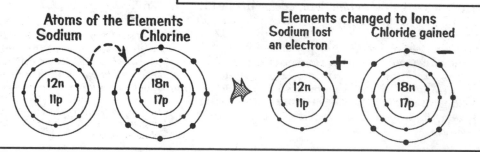

Atoms of the Elements
Sodium   Chlorine

Elements changed to Ions
Sodium lost   Chloride gained
an electron

exposed to negative energies of any kind long enough, the potential result will be detrimental to our health—physical, emotional, mental or spiritual.

Poisons, for example, change the relationship of neuron firing in the body and block out vast areas of the nervous system. Pesticides cause damage and mutation in the body by altering the process of transmission of genetic material, thereby changing how the body is run by its own DNA. Consequently, if we eat a food that has been sprayed with pesticides, our chances of forming mutant cells is greater than if we do not. Furthermore, the danger for us is not as great as it is for other generations that come after us.

As we begin to explore how the energies of the chakras interact in the auric field and the effect of these energies on the body's processes, we begin to see how these energies control the growth and function of each part of the body.

There was a time in this country when it was believed that to be without a certain body part meant one would never have a particular bodily function again. During the 1950's and 1960's people who had gallbladder surgery were told they would never again be able to eat normally. Yet there are many people in this country without gallbladders who somehow manage to digest food. What does that mean? It means that they have so much energy in the gallbladder area that the body, even with less bile, continues to break down food. Consequently, those without gallbladders still digest food. In other words, the organ itself is not as important as the energy that produces it. Not the organ, not the cell, but energy is the basic component of the body.

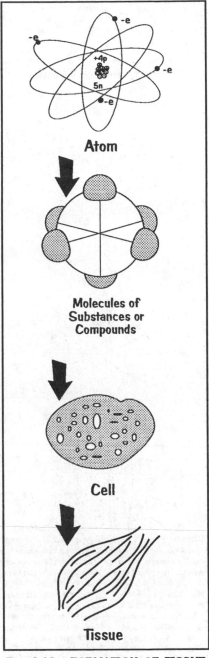

Atom

Molecules of Substances or Compounds

Cell

Tissue

Fig. 3.10. FORMATION OF TISSUE. Atoms combine to create molecules of different substances or compounds. These combine to create more complex compounds which then combine to create cells. Cells then differentiate to form a multitude of tissue types. Computer drawing by M.M. Smith/ Techni-Visions

65

Identical Nature of the Chakras

Existing literature on the chakras,[53] indicates the necessity to have "open" chakras. A chakra in actuality cannot be opened; it cannot be closed. Nevertheless these terms are frequently used to indicate a greater or lesser amount of energy which is actually being produced by a particular chakra at a particular time. In relation to this, a chakra may be "blocked" wherein the energy flow is restricted. In any case, however, a chakra is always there; it is always spinning. It turns the way it wants to turn based on its particular viewpoint of reality.

As previously noted, each chakra has its own particular point of view. However, according to Hermetic tradition, all the chakras are essentially identical.[54] Our research[55] showed them to be the same size. Each is basically the same shape. Most importantly, each chakra has, if not an essence of all the other chakras, at least a matrix or network that allows for another chakra to exist. The first chakra, for instance does not particularly care whether there are any other chakras. That state of consciousness is content to be, in and of itself. However, there is a network that allows for "other" (the viewpoint of the second chakra) contained in it. Simply stated, each chakra is both unique and potentially interactive with each other chakra, having both a specific viewpoint and the structure for a distinctly different one.

What this network means in terms of treatment of disease is that if an individual had a problem or an illness, it would not matter which chakra center a healer focused on; the problem would be solved if the healer

[53] See notes 25 and 41, Part One Chapter Two. H.P. Blavatsky, *The Secret Doctrine*, op. cit., also contains information on the seven chakras. More contemporary works are Walter J. Kilmer, *The Human Aura*, New Jersey: Citadel Press, 1965; Hiroshi Motoyama, with Rande Brown, *Science and the Evolution of Consciousness: Chakras, Ki, and Psi*, Brookline, Massachusetts: Autumn Press, Inc., 1978 (as well as Motoyama's *Theories of the Chakras*, op. cit.); and David Tansley, *The Raiment of Light: A Study of the Human Aura*, New York: Methuen, Inc., Arcana Division, 1987.

[54] This is implied in the main tenet of Hermetism: "As above, so below." (See Volume Four).

[55] The Rolf Study. Cf. Appendix.

treated any one chakra long enough because all the others would bounce into alignment. When people say to me, "What about the healer who is so insensitive that he's been treating your third chakra when your problem's really in the first?" I tell them, "The healing might still be effective, for in focusing on the third chakra, the first is forced to function."

Location of the Chakras

The seven major chakras are located along a central axis parallel to the spinal column of the physical body (see Fig. 3.11). Furthermore, each of the chakras has a traditional placement. The placement of the first chakra is between the base of the spine and the pubic bone. The second chakra is situated behind and just below the navel. The third chakra should sit in the V formed by the ribcage; however, in most Americans the third center is displaced to the left so that its location is closer to the pancreas than to the center of the body. (The reasons for this displacement will be further discussed in Volume Three.) The fourth center, or heart chakra, is situated midway between the two breasts, while the fifth chakra is located at the throat. The sixth chakra, also referred to as the third eye, is located between the brows, and the seventh, or crown chakra, which faces upward, is located at the top of the head. The first three chakras are often termed the "lower chakras" or the "lower centers", the fourth chakra, the "transitional" or the "transformational center", and the upper three chakras referred to as the "upper chakras" or the "upper centers".

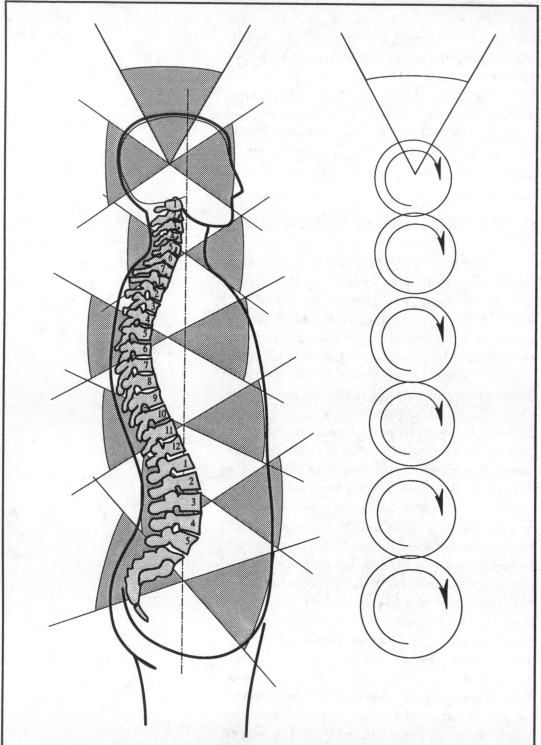

Fig. 3.11.   LOCATION OF THE CHAKRAS IN RELATION TO THE BACKBONE AND
THE FRONT OF THE BODY.
Computer drawing by M.M. Smith/Techni-Visions.

The Flow
of Energy Up the Chakras

When a stimulus comes into the body it is registered in the first chakra. The response is a change in the electromagnetic field of the first chakra, producing an energy flow out of the first center, into the second,

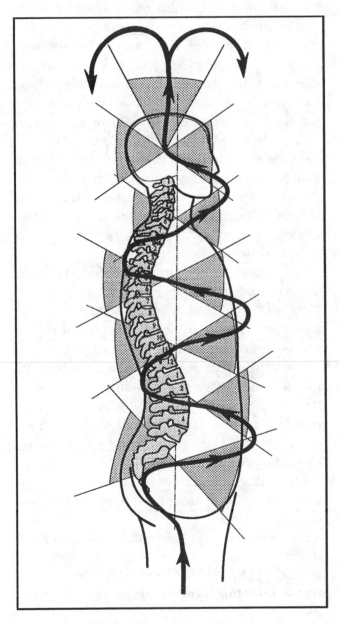

Fig. 3.12. FLOW OF ENERGY UP THE CHAKRAS. Computer drawing by M.M. Smith/Techni-Visions.

out the third, and into the heart chakra. In many of us the heart chakra is typically the place where this flow of energy is absorbed or drained from the field. The heart chakra is also one of the main locations of tension in the body; neck and shoulder problems start in the back of the heart chakra as well. However, if energy is not drained or absorbed when it enters the heart center, it is then free to continue out the fifth chakra, in the sixth and finally out the seventh or crown chakra.

That process of in and out, in and out, in and out becomes important. The source of the energy that moves throughout the body is the earth's magnetic field, acted upon and modified by the electrical field of that body. Other philosophical points of view propose that the source of this energy is the universe above. However, it is my experience that it is the earth's magnetic field which is the major source of the energy that flows in and out our chakra system, wherein it is acted upon either to our benefit or detriment.

When energy enters the body through our feet and moves up to the first chakra, it does so by moving from our thighs in the direction of our tailbone, which spins the energy down and forward at an angle (see Fig. 3.12). Thus, the first chakra does not really face forward. We are essentially sitting on it. Neither is it really like the crown, which is parallel to the surface of the earth and perpendicular to the remaining five chakras. In meditation we are always told to keep our spines straight, but flexible. This is so we can move around and locate the angle of the first chakra.

When energy leaves the first chakra, it is then drawn into the second. It enters the second chakra below the navel—most of us have a little roll of fat where energy enters the second center—and then it angles back and hits the waist (see Fig. 3.12). Thus the angle of the energy flow is low in the front but high in the back.

Next, the energy flows up the spine and out the back of the adrenal cortex, where the third chakra pulls it forward (see Fig. 3.12). At that point, most Americans pull the energy to the left toward the pancreas, and from there energy flows out. The heart chakra then has to work harder to pull it back in. Much of the problem that our culture has in "opening" the heart chakra is a result of the loss of energy in its movement from the left side over toward the heart center. If energy were allowed to flow directly up the center of the body, as it should, then the heart chakra would have a better opportunity to gather that energy mass and bring it back in more easily.

As energy leaves the heart chakra, it exits through the back of the heart center, bounces off the spine, projecting itself forward, whereupon it is drawn into the thymus (see Fig. 3.12). After reaching the thymus, the energy then flows upward and through the thymus to pass through the voice box where it can be manifested as speech (see Fig. 3.12).

Energy then continues to flow into the sixth chakra, also called the third eye. From antiquity this center has been cloaked in "mystery". Nearly everyone would agree that there is nothing mysterious about physical sight: the eyes see. For some, psychic sight may seem mysterious, but it is not. The third eye also sees; it allows us several kinds of perceptions. It provides the means by which we perceive extrasensorily. It should also enable us to see *what is so*, not just what is ours. We as a people tend to "see" or "take in" what is in our own energy flow, what is

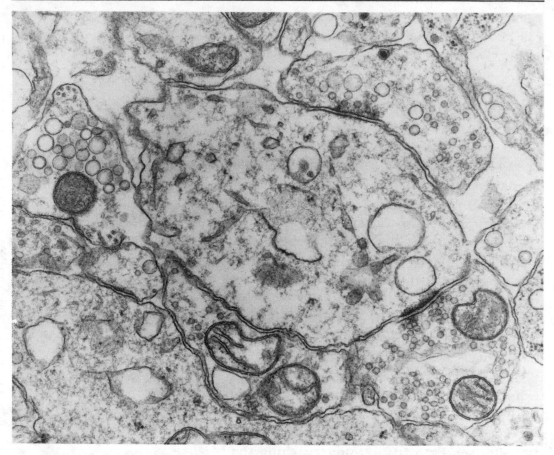

Fig. 3.13. SYNAPSE. Two axons terminating on a dendrite. The dendrite is the large cell in the middle surrounded by axons. Synaptic vesicles carry neuron transmitters. Omicron/Photo Researchers, Inc.

56 This pattern holds if energy is allowed to flow up and out. However, if one chooses to do anything with the energy, the flow will reflect off the pineal and then hit the pituitary, after which it will continue its movement out through the third eye, where manifestation can occur. The ancient Egyptians symbolized this movement in their image of a cobra poised and ready to strike, head expanded. This image can be found in several Egyptian temple reliefs, such as that of Sethos I at Abydos.

57 "At the top of the head (The Brahman Gate), or at Mahabatin, there are one thousand petals." (*Yoga Chudamani Upanishad*, v. 6.)

reflected from our own field, what is on our own path. We do not often see a complete picture but instead focus on individual rather than universal problems. Thus, we continue to "see through a glass darkly." (I Corinthians 13:12) The third eye allows us a clearer, more expansive vision.

After entering the third eye, the energy flow touches the pituitary gland,[56] reflects off the pineal gland and mushrooms out through the top of the crown (see Fig. 3.12). The seventh chakra is often referred to as the Diamond Sutra or the Diamond Lotus or the Thousand-petaled Lotus.[57] In fact, there are many neurological synapses here.

The auric field has a movement that tends to make energy "sweeps" which are

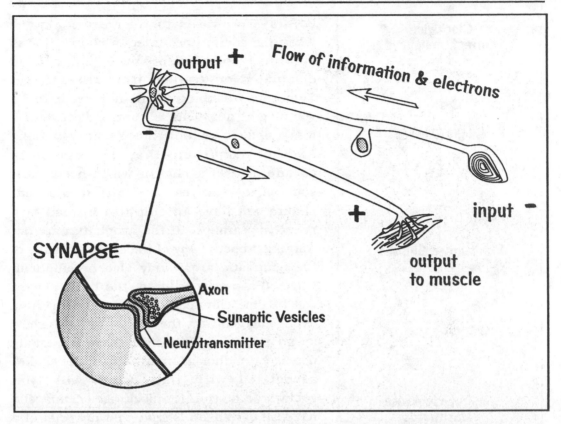

output **+**

Flow of information & electrons

−

input **−**

output
to muscle

SYNAPSE

Axon

Synaptic Vesicles

Neurotransmitter

usually about three or four inches apart. For example, the energy from the foot circles around the ankle, back through the calf, out through the knee and so on through the body. This serpentine dance of the auric field through the body and chakras produces a very complex interaction with the body's neurological and physiological systems.

Direction of Spin of the Chakras

When energy enters the body it moves upward from one chakra to the next. In some cases, however, this energy can be lost before traversing all the chakras. Generally a healthy, functioning chakra will spin or turn in a clockwise direction (when we are viewing the front of a person), so that the energy will

Fig. 3.14. FUNCTION OF A SYNAPSE. The synapse provides the connection between nerve cells (neurons). The axon is the output side where synaptic vesicles remain ready to carry information through the neurotransmitter to the receiving side which may be another axon, a cell or a dendrite. Neurotransmitters can either inhibit or excite response in the nervous system. The number of synapses within the brain and spinal cord directly affect our ability to integrate and modify sensory input and experiential memory so as to achieve a desired motor response. Computer drawing by M.M. Smith/ Techni-Visions.

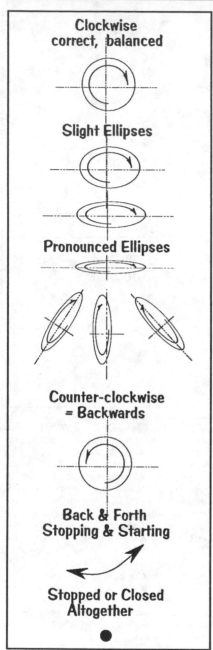

Clockwise
correct, balanced

Slight Ellipses

Pronounced Ellipses

Counter-clockwise
= Backwards

Back & Forth
Stopping & Starting

Stopped or Closed
Altogether

Fig. 3.15. DIRECTION OF CHAKRA SPIN.

58 This is true above the equator. Healthy chakras spin counterclockwise below the equator.

59 More specifically, a crystal is able to rectify the moving electromagnetic field of the chakra into a direct current. See p. 97 Chapter Four for a discussion of direct and alternating currents.

be drawn upwards to the next chakra.[58] When the energy encounters a chakra that is spinning counterclockwise, it will be dissipated or drained from the system. Sometimes a chakra will not seem to be spinning at all. This is often indicative of a weak chakra, which blocks energy flow. Another condition that is sometimes encountered is a chakra with an elliptical spin. If the pancreas is damaged, the third chakra will have an elliptical instead of a round appearance. If the lymphatics are not working properly, any of the chakras in any of the lymphatic areas may also be elliptical. Often, if a person is tired, the heart chakra will become elliptical. If there is something wrong energetically, the chakra will also show as an ellipse. If, however there is serious damage or pathology in any organ, the chakra associated with that organ will spin backwards or counter-clockwise. Thus, the *direction of rotation, shape,* and *diameter* of a chakra indicates the state of its energy and the health of its corresponding or adjacent physical organs. Some healers actually see this movement in much the same way as they see an aura; others feel it or sense it tactilely or empathetically within their own bodies.

When used as a pendulum, a prism or crystal is a tool that can corroborate chakra movement. This is because a crystal is an effective energy transmitter.[59] When a crystal is suspended over the chakra of a reclining person, the energy of the spinning chakra will cause the crystal to swing in a corresponding motion. The kind of movement in the chakra will be duplicated in the movement of the crystal: circular, clockwise, counterclockwise, elliptical, or sometimes even flat (back and forth).

There is another important explanation for the backwards movement of a chakra. The moon cycle or menstrual cycle causes a woman's central meridian to reverse direction for nine days of the month. During this time some of her chakras, usually every other one, turn backwards. This is not necessarily indicative of damage or illness. This time of the month is a sloughing-off period, an elimination cycle, which is also intended to eliminate concepts, ideas and bad feelings along with any impurities expelled with the flow of blood.

Men as well as women have this twenty-eight day cycle. While the male cycle is not a physiological one, it is one of regeneration in much the same way as is a woman's cycle. Culturally men are not taught to take advantage of that regenerative cycle. During these times, both men's and women's energy flow actually reverses, as may their chakras. For purposes of procreation, ideally the couple's cycles of downward energy flow should occur simultaneously.[60]

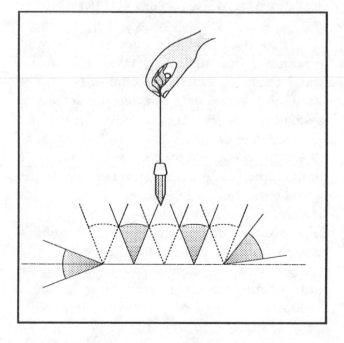

Fig. 3.16. PENDULUM. A crystal pendulum can be used to check the direction of spin of the chakra.

[60] The moon cycle and its effects on both men and women will be further discussed in Volume Two.

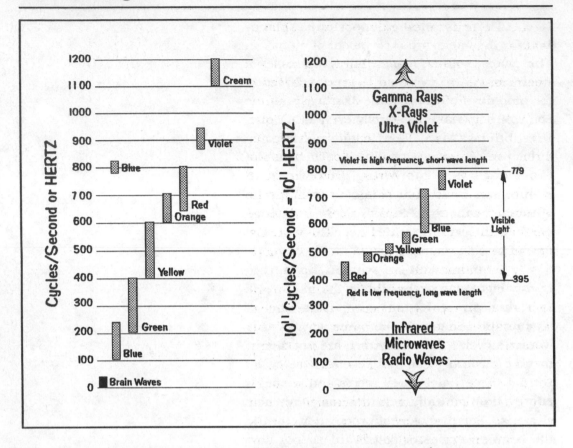

Fig. 3.17. AURIC AND VISIBLE LIGHT. Frequencies recorded from The Rolf Study as compared to the frequencies of visible light. Computer drawing from Rolf Study data by M.M. Smith/Techni-Visions.

Changing Frequencies: Interaction Between Chakras

In discussing the chakras we have to remember that although it is interesting theoretically to think of a chakra in and of itself, no person exists through the activity of a single chakra. Each of us exists through an interaction of many chakras. By focusing our attention on one chakra center or another, we limit ourselves to a single viewpoint of the world. Nothing really ever happens *in* a chakra. A chakra is only a point of origin. It is the effect of energy moving *through* a chakra which is important. Where a flow of energy (a sensory impression, an idea and so on) encounters the energy of a spinning chakra, it is pulled upward. It is this dynamic which moves energy from chakra to chakra.

As it spins, each chakra—a unique electromagnetic wave generator—creates a particular frequency. The frequency generated appears as a color that is unique only to that chakra. Since each chakra emits a different color, we should ideally have all colors present in our auras. However, as a culture we Americans somehow manage to take seven individual chakra colors and make them all into one color, yellow. This curious and unhealthy phenomenon is examined more closely in Volume Three.

When the system is functioning appropriately, there is a specific mathematical relationship between the frequencies of the chakras: the frequency of each chakra increases as we move up the chakra system. Not only was this found to be so in the lab,[61] but this phenomenon is discussed in the *Veda* and in other ancient texts, where it is referred to as "the multiple".[62]

This change in frequency makes possible the separation of different states of consciousness. There is a jump between the physical tactility of the first chakra and feelings in the second chakra; a greater jump between those feelings and the opinions of the third chakra; and a leap between those opinions and second feelings in the heart center. Thus, as the energy moves through the body it undergoes numerous complex modifications through the repeated increase of frequency. This allows for a kind of complexity that we probably do not think about but take for granted.

[61] Cf. Appendix.

[62] Cf. note 25 Part One Chapter Two.

Relationships Between the Chakras

Intake and Output

Chakras relate to other chakras in various ways. One of these relationships is that of *polarity*. A chakra can be *positive* (+) or *negative* (-). Those chakras which move energy out the front of the body are called *output* chakras and have a positive polarity. Those into which energy flows are called *intake* chakras and have negative polarity. Each chakra with a given polarity is connected to the remaining chakras of the same polarity. For example, energy flowing up the chakra system into the fourth chakra (intake) will immediately connect to the second and sixth chakras (which are also intake chakras). Thus, the upper chakras of each polarity have access to the lower chakras of the same polarity and vice versa.

In addition to polarity, the respective functions—intake and output—are interrelated. Having an opinion in the third chakra is connected to the fifth chakra (speech, expression) because one speaks an opinion. The second, fourth and sixth centers (which are intake centers) form one relationship, and chakras one, three, five and seven (which are output centers) form another relationship. In most instances, one intake chakra will connect with the other two corresponding intake chakras, and an output chakra will connect with two of its corresponding output centers. If we want to make changes, we will energize the active or output chakras in combination so that we are moving concepts or changes through them. On the other hand, if we want to maintain a pleasant feeling, or one that is familiar or comfortable,

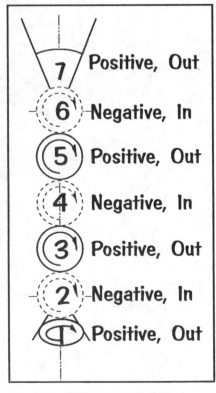

Fig. 3.18. CHAKRA POLARITY.

7 Positive, Out
6 Negative, In
5 Positive, Out
4 Negative, In
3 Positive, Out
2 Negative, In
1 Positive, Out

we usually energize chakras two, four and six. By energizing certain chakras and not others, then, our experience is affected.

Color Opposites, Color Therapy and Empowering with Opposites

Probably the oldest text that discusses chakra colors is the *Upanishads*, and although there is some disparity among authors regarding the specific colors associated with individual chakras, the rainbow spectrum of chakra colors is generally agreed upon. If we look then at the traditional seven chakras, the first chakra is red; the second radiates orange; the third is yellow; the fourth, green; the fifth radiates blue; the sixth is violet; and the seventh chakra is white. In discussing the major chakra centers and their colors, we must keep in mind that our chakras are not necessarily these colors at any time in our lives; these are,however, the colors they ought to be all the time.

Just as the chakras are related by means of their opposite functions (input and output), they also share a relationship of opposite or complementary colors. Interestingly, these color complements do not correspond to those of the light spectrum, but more closely (although not completely) duplicate the color complements of pigment. Most people who have had a basic art class recognize pigment color opposites or complements. By definition, the primary colors are red, yellow and blue; secondary colors are orange, green and purple or violet.

Each of the secondary colors is a complement of a particular primary color and vise versa. A secondary color is made by blending equal portions of two primary colors. Specifically, when two primaries are mixed to

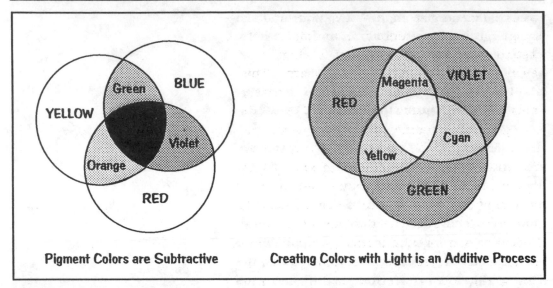

Pigment Colors are Subtractive

Creating Colors with Light is an Additive Process

Fig. 3.19. ADDITIVE AND SUB-TRACTIVE COLOR SYSTEMS. Three pools of light (cyan, magenta, yellow) overlap on a white screen in the additive color mixing process. Pigments use the primaries—red, blue and yellow—in the subtractive color system to obtain secondary colors. The mixture of all three primary colors results in black, the absence of light, as the consequence of blocking out or subtracting all wave lengths; in contrast, additive color mixing combines colors to produce white light. In other words, pigments absorb, while light reflects.

form a secondary color, that secondary color is the complement of the remaining primary. The inverse is also true. Green (a blend of yellow and blue primaries) is the complement of red as red is also green's complement. Orange and blue are complementary, and yellow and violet are the remaining complementary colors.

When treating an illness by healing with energies, an imbalance of any one color can be treated, corrected and enhanced with its opposite or complementary color: a primary color is usually treated with its opposite secondary color; a secondary color imbalance is usually treated with its primary opposite. Actually the most common choice is to treat an excess of red (as in pain or inflammation) with green.

Someone suffering from an emotional trauma, for instance, would have a large orange auric field. By channeling blue into the second chakra, emotions can be calmed and brought under control. On the other hand, if someone were not able to express one's self emotionally, the auric field would be predominately blue. In this case we would want to remove the blue and replace it with orange. Take, for example, a specific case in which a healer is working with a client who has not cried in seven or eight years. This client has probably gone through a severe depression or trauma and decided never to feel again. By channeling orange energy, the client can begin the process of crying and releasing in an atmosphere of safety and support. Where analytical skills and memory recall are required, an abundance of yellow is necessary in the aura. On the other hand, there are times when there is an over-abundance of yellow. We might become entangled in mental "chatter" or find ourselves replaying the same ideas or rationalizations over and over again. To stop this "chatter", the violet frequency from the third eye needs to be added to the aura. This more creative color, which enables people to visualize, shuts down the yellow, bringing the mental loop to a stop.

These are only some of the uses of color opposites. As healers, whenever we treat one center, we also have to treat its opposite. If someone has a sore throat or a loss of voice (as is so common in the consciousness movement), the problem is a shortage of blue (fifth chakra). Because emotions and expression are interrelated, however, the orange center (second chakra) must also be treated.

Furthermore, certain organs respond specifically to certain colors. Generally, an organ will respond to the color (frequency) of the chakra in which it is located and also to the color (frequency) of the opposing or complementary chakra. For example, the pancreas, which is located in the mid-body behind the stomach, sits in the third chakra.

The native frequency of the third chakra is yellow. The pancreas will respond to both yellow and to its complementary color, violet, the native frequency of the sixth chakra. These colors would be used to rebalance energies of the organ and thus to initiate healing and regeneration of the organ as required.

Each chakra, in fact, contains both its primary color and its color opposite. The throat chakra (the fifth center), for example, contains both blue and orange, while its opposite or complementary center, the second chakra, contains orange and blue. However, in the case of the second chakra the blue is absorbed and in the case of the throat chakra the orange is absorbed. These absorbed frequencies represent the passive side of each respective chakra and thus the opposite or complementary function. In other words, the orange in the second chakra is predominant and the blue is the power behind it, while in the fifth chakra, the orange is the power behind the blue. Each chakra contains its opposite component which helps empower it. For instance, in order to speak (blue) effectively, we must have full abdominal breath (orange), and in order to breathe fully (green), our hips (red) must be open.

Whatever color is channeled into the body will be sorted or filtered in an appropriate manner by each chakra. As the energy moves up the chakra system, each chakra takes the energy being received and sorts out the particular color (frequency) needed in that area of the body.

A widely used practice among healers is to channel white light. It is true that all colors are contained within the white frequency. However, always channeling white is perhaps the worst use and waste of healing energy; white is not what the body particularly needs. If it needs a specific color, such as violet, and only white is channeled, the body then has to go through the process of filtering out violet from the white.

In certain situations, however, white is an advantageous color for a healer to use. When a client is talking his energy out faster than the healer can put it in, by channeling white, the healer can force the client to "leave his body". The client thus goes into an altered state of consciousness in which his mind is quiet. The healer can then begin to work on the body to affect the needed changes.

The theory of color and color opposites relates to another very important concept, that of paradox. Anytime we say something is so, and something else is not so simply because it opposes or seems to contradict the first idea, we are negating the universal experience of paradox. It is often the case that one thing is so and another is probably so as well. If we are too quick to resolve things because we are looking at them from only one point of view, then we cannot begin inclusive thinking nor learn to "hold paradox". The chakra system is balanced. It represents not just one level of reality, not just one viewpoint, but several. One chakra does not simply "oppose" another; it is also the other's "complement": it *completes* the other. The interaction of chakras is the entire process. All must function together in balance in order for each and every person to function as a *complete* sentient being.

The Male, Female, Androgyny and Exogeny in The Chakras

Historically, chakras have been described as having *masculine* and *feminine* characteristics. The positive polarity or output function of a chakra tends *to push* energy out or through the system, while the negative polarity or intake function tends to *attract*, to *draw in*, to *pull*. In Oriental philosophy, positive-masculine energy is termed "yang", and negative-feminine energy, "yin". (Refer to Volume Two for a discussion of Yin and Yang.) Ordinarily the function of the first chakra is viewed as being masculine or male; it pushes energy out. The second chakra's function tends to be feminine or female; it pulls in. Thereafter, these functions alternate: the third, fifth and seventh chakras are male, and the fourth and sixth are female.

There is another more exact way to look at these functions. We can view them as: masculine, feminine, androgynous, feminine, masculine, androgynous, exogenous. In other words, the first chakra's vitality is very yang. The emotion of the second is very yin. The intellect component of the third chakra is both masculine and feminine; it is androgynous. The transformative property of the heart chakra is feminine, while the response/expression of the throat center is masculine. The wisdom factor and creative aspect of the sixth chakra is androgynous. Finally, when realization is attained in the seventh chakra, we are exogenous; we are out of the system. We are neither male nor female, nor are we androgynous; we are transformed, we are realized, we are complete.

Fig. 3.20. CHAKRA FUNCTIONS.

Exogenous
Androgynous
Masculine
Feminine
Androgynous
Feminine
Masculine

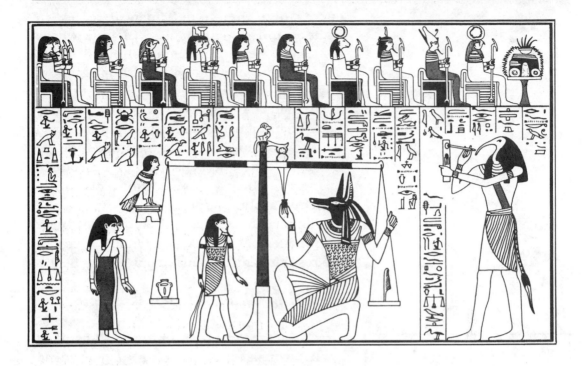

Sustaining a Balanced Energy Field

Maintaining Constancy

All of the spiritual disciplines teach us to be consistent with energy. The ancient "Egyptian Negative Confessions" or "Recensions" from the *Book of Ani*,[63] the *Noble Eightfold Path* of the Buddhists,[64] the *Dharma Sastras*[65] and Yogic practices of the Hindus, the *Torah* of Judaism and the *Ten Commandments* of Judaism and Christianity are all intended to instruct one in the ways of maintaining consistency in life and thus sustaining a balanced energy field. Take, for example, the commandment "Thou shalt not covet thy neighbor's goods." If we "covet" or ardently desire another's possession, that desire is going to cause a fluctuation in our energy; specifically, we are going to take an

Fig. 3.21. THE WEIGHING OF THE HEART FROM THE EGYPTIAN BOOK OF THE DEAD. Ani's soul (left) awaits the decision of the weighing of his heart (left balance) against the feather of Maat or Justice (right balance). Thoth (right) records the results of the weighing, while Anubis tests the tongue of the balance.

[63] The *Book of Ani* is the 125th chapter of the Egyptian *Book of the Dead*. Cf. note 33, Part One Chapter Two. The "negative confessions" were spoken before Osiris at the time of one's judgment (the weighing of the heart), prior to resurrection.

[64] The *Eightfold Path* consists of right views, right intention, right speech, right conduct, right livelihood, right effort, right mindfulness, and right concentration. Following this path, according to Buddhist teachings, is the way to stop desiring and thus suffering, since suffering is a result of one's desires for pleasure, power and continued existence.

[65] The *Dharma-Sastras* along with the *Dharma Sutras* contain rules of conduct, rites and expiations as well as the doctrine of karma or karman and the definition of dharma. Hindu law in the judicial sense is completely embedded in religious law and practice. (*Encyclopaedia Britannica*, Vol. 20, 1985, p. 590).

energy dive that is detrimental to us, in addition to being harmful to the one whose possession we desire. Such a strong desire is obviously inconsistent with spiritual goals in any religious discipline. Such energy fluctuation is unhealthy to our physical being. Each energy fluctuation causes pathology in the body because it creates so huge a dip in the field that our cells do not reproduce properly, blood does not circulate appropriately, plaque builds up in the cardiovascular system and so on. All these are functions of inconsistency in our lives and the resulting fluctuations in our energy field.

Avoiding Chakra Displacement

In the American culture, a result of such inconsistency is *chakra displacement.* The chakra system is designed to function in a particular way. When all the centers are aligned and functioning appropriately, a healthy process occurs. When information enters the chakra system, it comes up through the feet and legs (the secondary "feeder" centers) and is recorded as a concept in the first chakra. Then, as it progresses up through the remaining chakras, we have a feeling [in the second chakra], an opinion [in the third center], a second feeling [in the fourth chakra], a response [in the fifth center], an insight [in the sixth chakra], and a release [in the seventh center]. This healthy alignment, however, does not often occur.

As was previously noted, Americans in particular displace the third chakra to the left. Americans are top-heavy. We are not *well-grounded.* In meditation, if we bring energy down from above, we often do not bring it all the way to the ground, nor do we bring it all the way up and out through the

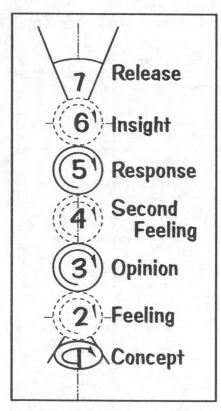

Fig. 3.22. *CHAKRA ALIGNMENT. Aligned chakras process in a healthy way.*

top of our heads when we bring energy up from the earth. Some people have actually succeeded in blocking all energy flow below the waist. As a result, all the chakras are displaced upwards by two steps: the first chakra sits where the third should be, the second chakra is where the fourth should be, and so on. Consequently, our first chakra consciousness and our intellect become mixed up; we begin to think that concept, not intellect, originates in the third chakra. In other words, we think concept begins with the intellect; and thus we believe that concepts do not exist outside of ourselves.

This brings us to a very important point. Things *are* or *are not*, actually and in fact, in spite of what we think or believe. Our belief in something, however, may bring it into existence or our denial exclude it from our reality. That is, we may actually be able to successfully block certain things from our consciousness through a process of progressive amnesia; but it requires that we expend a great amount of energy to suppress the reality around us.

This blocking and suppression is exactly what happens when chakras become displaced. (Sometimes this is called neurosis.) This occurs because first feeling is (mis)placed in the heart, opinion in the throat, second feeling then gets mixed up with our intuition, and consequently, there can be no release. A headache is a typical physical response to this. In fact, we should always check when we feel a headache coming on to see if we have this displacement, because often that is what has happened. This check can be done by simply observing and feeling if the lower body and hips are cold or numb. If so, the indication is that energy flow is absent and has likely been displaced. One of the body's responses to stress, hypertension, is a more life-threatening result of this displacement. It is my experience that prolonged displacement of the chakras will ultimately lead to some form of pathology.

This brings up a very important question. If it is so unhealthy, how does anyone avoid displacing? We start by knowing we have a place in our body upon which we are sitting. This requires that we become aware of the lower centers and of our breathing. Breathing into the lower centers is very helpful; it breaks the displacing pattern. Proper grounded meditation is also effective. A researcher at U.C. Berkeley reported that people who meditate longer than three years actually develop a different way of thinking and do not revert back to their old way.[66] Though one has to meditate for three years or more for that change finally to take place, the change, which is not big, but slow and subtle, requires only ten or twenty minutes a day.

Meditation is one way to avoid chakra displacement. Once displacement occurs, however, one must also have a method for realigning the chakras. Alignment means being centered within, and chakra alignment itself is the means for sustaining a balanced energy field. Chakras are aligned primarily through a physical process.

In the East, a spiritual student is first taught a physical discipline so that the chakras line up and the body can feel the place where one chakra turns against another. In fact, what one feels is the heat generated at each intersection or junction where one rotating chakra encounters another.

Generally, we do not feel this heat until someone positions our bodies in such a way as to align the chakras. In Oriental

[66]   Refer to Elaine and Arthur Aron, *The Maharishi Effect, A Revolution Through Meditation*, Walpole, New Hampshire: Stillpoint Publishing, 1986.

disciplines this is done by a Master. In Buddhism, this is usually done by striking the meditating student on the appropriate areas of the back with a stick. Eventually we have to learn to move, bend and sit until we find this kind of alignment without assistance. When we have achieved this, we may experience our bodies as having "a core".

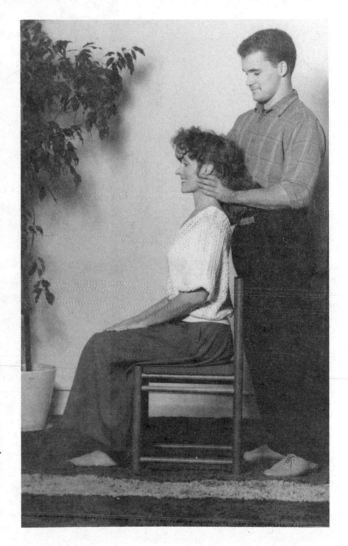

Fig. 3.23. ALIGNMENT EXERCISE. Photo by Susan Rothschild.

Alignment Exercise

For those of you who do not have this physical sense of what it means to be centered "on your core", there is an exercise that can be done with a partner to experience what chakra alignment feels like (see Fig. 3.23). Sit down in a chair with your spine straight, knees bent, feet flat on the floor. Have your partner pull you straight up gently by the head; that should bring you into alignment. Try to feel movement (vibration) at the hips and the heart and then up the whole core. Then you will begin to feel heat between the chakras. Another sensation you might notice, if you are sensitive to it, is a rush of energy out the crown chakra. If you can feel these things, you know you have achieved chakra alignment.

Chapter Four

THE CHAKRAS AND HEALING

Scanning the Body and Transmitting or Channeling Energy

Healers talk about *transmitting energy, running energy* or *channeling energy.* Sometimes the term *running current* will even be used.[67] These terms all refer to the same process. Several times in this volume there have been references to one of these phrases usually followed by a brief description or clarification. I now offer a more complete explanation of what it means to *transmit energy.*

Before healers lay hands on a person and begin to transmit energy, they should scan the client's body with their hands (see Fig. 4.1). Basically, this is the way most healers, especially those who have not yet developed any other psychic sense (such as seeing auras), obtain necessary information about blocks in energy flow, damaged chakras, and so on. The procedure is simple. The healer feels the edges of the client's aura by holding a hand some distance above the client's reclining body and moving the hand toward the client's body until there is a sense of contact, of presence. This contact often feels like a slight pushing sensation or a kind of bouyancy against the hand. Then the healer moves his hand along the edge of the

[67] Healer alert! Although these terms have been used interchangeably, please be aware that each denotes something specific. Running current, because of its specific scientific reference, is probably not an acceptable phrase to use. Again, while it is true that healers do act as channels in energy work, channeling energy may not be the most appropriate term to describe the energy process either, because of the connection of the term "channeling" to mediumship. My own preference in describing the energy process is to refer to it as the transmission or transference of energy.

Fig. 4.1. *SCANNING THE AURA.*
Photos by Susan Rothschild.

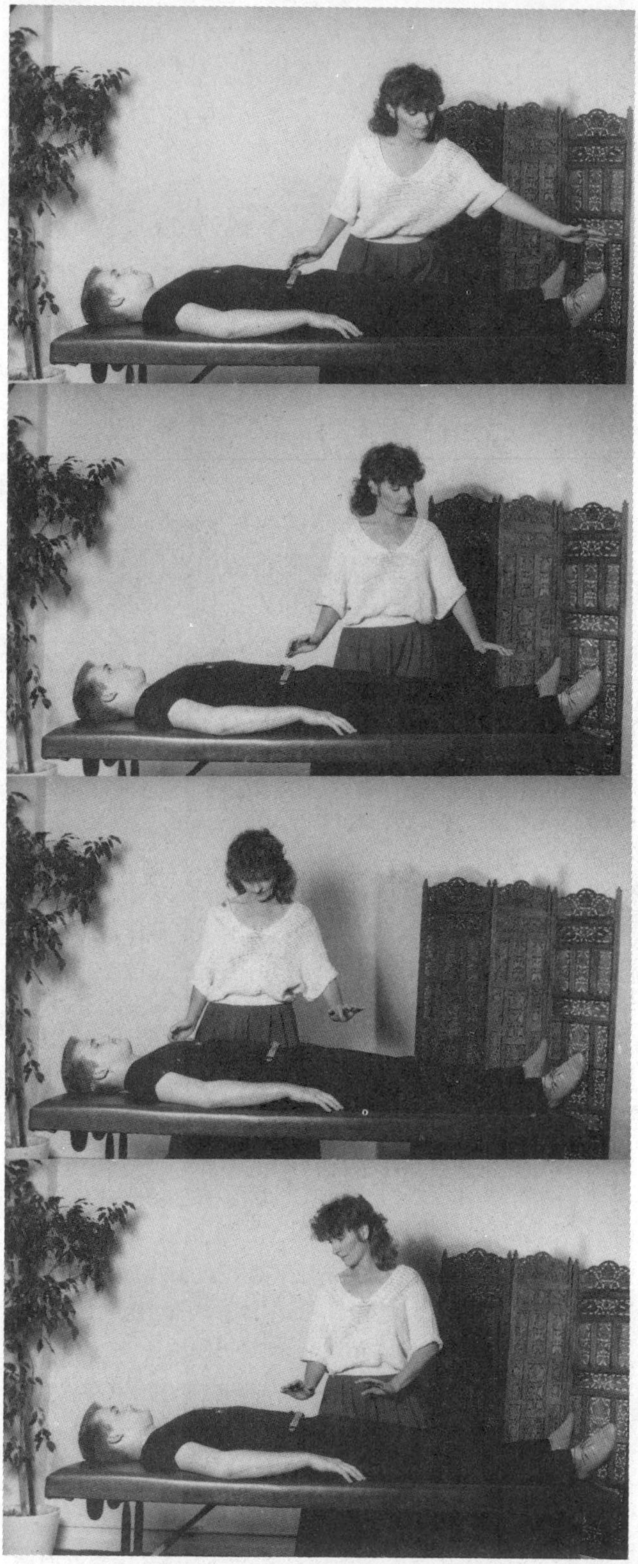

1.

2.

3.

4.

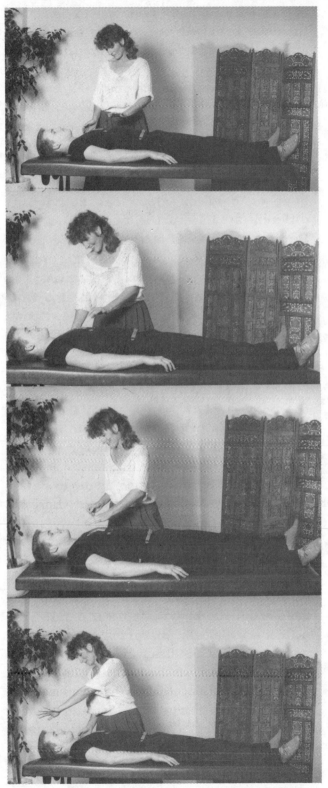

5.

6.

7.

8.

client's aura, usually from feet to head. As the hand is moved, the healer tries to sense any unusual or irregular phenomena at the outer edge or within the client's aura. Every part of the body feels different, but basically there should be a liquid-like sensation beneath the healer's hand. There should be a sense of flow. When one feels a "gap", "hole" or "bulge", one knows something is potentially wrong. Often the sensation is one of localized heat or cold or electrical activity as differentiated from the rest of the aura. During this process of scanning, the healer may ask questions of the client's present conditions or past injuries or traumas. The information that the healer obtains from scanning the aura, along with the client's own complaints, provides the healer with some idea of what needs to be healed: what organs are damaged, what chakras are unbalanced.

Any of us who heal should first scan the body—feel the aura—to discover the problem areas before beginning to transmit energy. After channeling energy into the client for a period of time, the healer needs to feel or scan the aura once again to obtain feedback on what the channeled energy is doing.

The actual process of *transmitting* or *channeling* energy is based on the electromagnetic nature of the body. Although it may have been known to the ancients, the facts about the body's electrical nature were neither scientifically known nor accepted until very recently. Specifically, electrical currents exist in parts of the body's nervous system. Everything electrical stems from the phenomenon of *charge* —positive and negative —which is measured in terms of electrons. A *negative charge* indicates a surplus of electrons, a *positive charge*, a scarcity of

Fig. 4.2. ELECTRICITY AND MAGNETISM. A further explanation of these phenomena appears on the following two pages.

•••••••••••*AS SCIENCE SEES IT*•••••••••••

ELECTRICITY

Electricity derives from the positive and negative charges within the atom and is basically a flow of negatively charged electrons. Because every atom contains both protons (+) and electrons (-) it is difficult to separate electricity from the physical properties of matter. In certain types of material, electrons become dislodged from the atom's outer shell. It is these free electrons that produce electrical current. Materials such as silver, copper and aluminum are good conductors because they contain a large number of free electrons that can bounce about from atom to atom. By contrast, insulative materials such as wood, glass or mica contain relatively few free electrons. In between the conductors are certain kinds of crystals which provide the medium for smaller currents. Free electrons behave chaotically until some form of energy causes the electrons to move in some direction. The free electrons are then guided from atom to atom in an orderly fashion. The influence which causes the electrons to move is called electromotive force or emf and is measured in volts. The current flow itself is measured in amperes (1 ampere = movement of 6.25×10^{18} electrons/second past a benchmark). The emf (V) is equal to the current (I) times the resistance (R) in the system. Energy to create an emf can be in any of several forms as listed below.

    a.   **Light.** Certain materials are particularly sensitive to light and actually generate their own emf when exposed to a light source. They convert light directly into electrical current. These materials are called photovoltaic cells or just photocells.

    b.   **Heat.** When two dissimilar metals are joined and one end heated, a current flows. This is known as a thermocouple and is used extensively in thermostats.

    c.   **Mechanical deformation of crystals.** Certain crystals have the ability to transform mechanical deformation into an emf. Tapping such a crystal with a hammer or bending it in one direction causes electrons to flow. When the bending stops, the current stops. Crystals with an orderly molecular structure, such as germanium and silicon, are called semiconductive and are the basis for piezoelectricity.

    d.   **Chemical.** By placing two dissimilar metals in a conducting solution, a flow of ions results and an ionic current is created. An example of this theory in use is the common automotive battery with its conductive solution of sulphuric acid. Sodium chloride and other ionic substances in aqueous solution also create the basis for an electrical current in water.

    e.   **Magnetic field.** An electric current can be created by an alternating or moving magnetic field. Generators and motors owe their complete operation to the use of this theory.

Some interesting research performed by Robert O. Becker and his associates has shown bones to behave like piezoelectric crystals and nerves to operate like direct current semiconductors. Becker postulated a primitive analog-coded information system, closely related to the nerves, which used semiconducting direct current. He further theorized that this system, either alone or together with the nerve impulse system, regulates growth, healing and other basic processes. Becker was able to reproduce the same kind of regenerating current which appeared naturally when salamander limbs were regrowing by implanting tiny batteries (silver and platinum wires separated by a resistor). The negative electrode was positioned at the wound in the bone marrow cavity. He found that the surrounding cells regenerated appropriately until they grew beyond the influence of the negative potential from the platinum electrode.

MAGNETISM

Magnetism relates to the direction of attraction and movement of particles. Electrical phenomena and magnetism are inseparable. The relationship between the two can be summarized in four fundamental laws referred to as Maxwell's equations, in tribute to his synthesis of electricity, magnetism and optics into one coherent theory.

1. **Coulomb's law** of electrostatics states that like charges repel and unlike charges attract with a force that increases as the two charges approach each other and decreases as the square of the distance between them increases.

2. Every **magnetic pole** is always accompanied by an opposite pole of equal strength.

3. **Ampere's law** states that an electric current flowing along a conductor is always accompanied by a magnetic field and the strength of this field increases as the size of the current increases. The field strength can be increased by winding the wire into a coil of many turns as shown in the figure below. A piece of iron placed in the center of the coil creates an electromagnet. This configuration is commonly used in solenoids.

4. **Faraday's law** describes the induction or creation of a current from a magnetic field. In addition, it states that a changing magnetic field is always accompanied by an electric field. The presence of a conductor is not required and the relation holds in empty space.

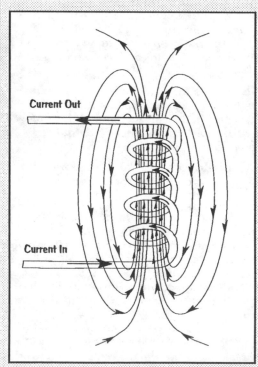

Current Out

Current In

Only weak magnets exist in nature. Black mineral ore, known as lodestone or magnetite, is able to pick up small bits of iron. To produce an artificial magnet, a piece of hard steel must be placed in an electric field. Especially strong magnets are produced by placing the steel in the center of a spiraling loop wire as shown in the figure to the left. It is interesting to note the similarity of this configuration to the kundalini force (electric current) and spinal column (magnetic field). In addition, the spiral of the DNA molecule shown in Fig. 3.8 also forms a similar shape.

For more complete explanations, see the Encyclopaedia Britannica, 15th Ed., Vol.18, 1985.

Computer drawing by M.M. Smith/Techni-Visions

them. Therefore an area becomes positively charged as electrons move out of it and negatively charged as electrons move into it. This flow of electrons is called a *current* which is measured in amperes (the amount of charge being moved). A *direct current* (DC) is a steady flow of electrons, while an *alternating current* (AC) is a back-and-forth flow. Most of our household appliances run on alternating current.

An *electric field* forms around any electric charge. The *electric field* is the space around a charged object in which an *electrical field potential* (positive or negative) can be detected. Any other charged object in the nearby field of the first object will be attracted (if their polarities are opposite) or repelled (if they are the same). This is the phenomenon of *magnetism*, and wherever an electrical field exists, there must also exist a magnetic field as well.

The significance of this for a healer is that any flow of electrons in the nervous system of the body sets up both an electric and a magnetic (electromagnetic) field around the current-carrying conductor (nerve fiber) which in turn affects other electrons nearby and ultimately the auric field. *Transmitting energy* actually refers to transmitting and maintaining a flow, a current of electrons. Direct current produces a stable electromagnetic field which in most cases is preferable to the unstable field created by alternating current (each time the current changes directions, the field collapses and reappears with its poles reversed).[68] The wonder and awesome reality of all this is that while both kinds of fields—electric and magnetic—decline with distance, their influence is theoretically infinite. Each time we as healers transmit energy into another,

[68] Whether electrons actually flow through the body of the healer into the client, or whether the healer produces a DC or AC potential that forces the electrons (already in the client's body) to move in accordance with the applied potential remains one of the major unanswered questions about the healing process. It is my hope that this question will be answered by future research.

the fields around us affect charged particles ever so slightly in the farthest galaxies.[69]

One of the results of the Rolf Study at UCLA was an audio aura-correlation sound tape.[70] I always recommend that my own healing students utilize this "aura" tape while they are learning to channel different colors (frequencies) of energy. It is somehow easier to channel a specific frequency by hearing its audio correlation than it is by trying to visualize it. Since purple is the frequency in which visualization occurs, what often happens when a particular color is visualized is that the color purple is channeled instead of the intended color. By using the audio-correlation tape and listening to the sound correlating to the specific color desired, the listener's body will begin to resonate at that frequency and in harmonics of that frequency, which can then be channeled. The ideal is, of course, for the healer to be able to discriminate tactilely the specific vibrations of individual colors of the energy being channeled. However, that is a very subtle process, and it usually takes a great deal of practice before it can be perfected.

Another process for transmitting energy is even more subtle. This is called channeling chakra to chakra. In other words, the healer channels from his or her own particular chakra into the corresponding chakra of a client. For example, if the person I am trying to heal has a heart problem, I can channel from my own heart chakra. It is true that the client and I may have different frequencies (or harmonics) of green in our hearts based on the harmonics that we tend to live in, but my green will mix quite well with the green in my client's heart since he has a heart problem and needs more green frequency. It must be remembered that our

---

69 Becker and Selden, op. cit., Chapter Four.

70 As of this writing, the audio-aura correlation sound tape, which was previously available through the Healing Light Center Church, has been removed from the market. It is my hope that Dr. Hunt will make this tape available again in the near future.

own chakras, in spite of us, have the capacity to make pure colors. Our own body, then, is our best guide to the spectrum of colors needed for the work healers do. By managing to isolate and sense the feeling of a specific vibration in a chakra, a pure color can be produced quite easily.

The actual sensation of transmitting energy is like flowing water, like a force moving through the healer's body. As an illustrative exercise let your arm drop and make yourself feel the arm at the tissue level. Do not visualize, do not mentalize the process. Just feel "water" coming up the body and running down the arm. Continue to concentrate on the flow down the arm until the pressure builds up in your hand. When you begin to sense a kind of movement, you know that the pressure is building up "in the hose". Then you are actually channeling. This is the feeling a healer has while running energy. The process requires concentration, but only at first. If one channels energy with any regularity, concentration is no longer necessary. Most healers can go on healing no matter what happens. The kids can come in, and the kittens go dashing across the dining room table with the kids hot after them. In the process of all this somebody asks for a peanut butter and jelly sandwich. An experienced healer will say, "Take the cat off the table; the peanut butter is in the cabinet", and not miss a beat of presence in the healer/client connection because running energy has become an athletic skill.

The more we channel and the more often we channel, the greater the muscle tone. If we channel very little, we do not have enough muscle tone to hold or run energy for any amount of time. Remember, the whole chakra and energy system is electromagnetic.

If there are no wires, there is no magnetism. Building more and more muscle tone provides the necessary energy-carrying capacity, and frequent channeling is what builds this muscle tone.

Exercise: Feeling Energy

The following exercise, for which you will need a partner, will assist you in experiencing the flow of energy and sensing what it feels like when two energy fields interact. Sit face to face with someone. Take hold of your partner's hand as though you were going to arm wrestle, but make a conscious effort to get palm chakra to palm chakra. That is the important part. Hold comfortably for about thirty seconds. Then pull your hand back so it is about six inches away from your partner's. What do you feel? Can you feel the "bouncing"? Take some time. Repeat the exercise. If it makes it easier for you to concentrate, close your eyes and focus your mind on your palm area, which is kind of cup shaped. Feel the "cup", put all of your consciousness into it and then move the focus so that your consciousness goes into your partner's hand. You may feel your energies pass as each of you moves into the other. Both of you are really transferring consciousness from your own hand into your partner's; you are actually merging.

Now ask yourself the question: Who has the better pulse? Just think about it. Decide whose pulse you like best, and then both of you adopt that one.

Next, slowly open your eyes. Move your hands apart about two inches. One of you should slowly move your hand while the other follows, staying in that field. Next, each

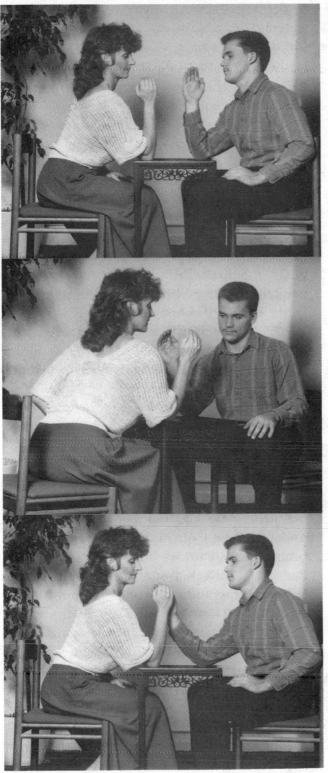

Fig. 4.4.   EXERCISE: FEELING ENERGY.   Photos   by   Susan Rothschild.

A.

Hold your partner's hand comfortably for about thirty seconds. Then pull your hand back so it is about six inches away from your partner's. What do you feel?

B.

Focus your mind on the palm area of your hand, which is cup shaped. Then slowly move your focus so your consciousness goes into your partner's hand. Try to feel the energies pass.

C.

Slowly move your hand while your partner follows, staying in your field. Then move your hand to one side out of that field. Then move your hand back into the field. Notice if you still feel a bond, a sense of mergence.

of you move your hand to one side out of that field. Then go back into it, and notice if you still feel that bond. Now, feel your partner's other hand. It should not feel the same. Then go back to the hand that shared the pulse. Examine it again.

The purpose of this exercise is to cause the hand to lose its normal sensing. Our normal sensing or our conscious feeling of the hand is either intake or output; what we do with our energy is either push or pull. In the above exercise you were forced to break your own boundary and merge with another. In that state of mergence you can sense the pulse, the strength of a heartbeat in another person. You knew which of the heartbeats felt better and were able to modulate accordingly.

Another purpose of this exercise is to acquire an understanding of how to approach a client. If we proceed from the outside without merging, even if we know the chakra system well, even if we know body symbology[71] as well as it can be known, we will come into the healing session with preconceived ideas about the meaning of somebody's illness and what the client's issues are. Therein we lose all of our sensitivity. We lose our own psychic process and invalidate ourselves before we really begin. If instead, we simply open or loosen and merge with that other body, the two of us have an experience of what "optimum" is for us both. Then there is an exchange of energies that prevents resistance patterns in the client. The intimacy of mergence at a full body level can be very threatening to people who are ill or who have never experienced that kind of intimacy with anyone before. Consequently, they may have many considerations about the whole healing process. However, if a healer "goes in" gently,

71   The human body speaks a symbolic language of health and disease, providing those who know how to listen with tools to restore a system to health. I often refer to this language as body symbology. Cf. note 148, Part Two, Chapter Six.

the client can slowly begin to experience merging and will then lower his defenses so the healing process can begin to work. It is a way of approach that is noninvasive.

Resistance to Being Healed

Occasionally I encounter someone who has made a conscious decision not to hear something, or an unconscious decision not to be healed. As you may already know, metaphysics teaches that if a person does not want a healing, he can reject it. The real resistance people have to the healing process working is that it changes their structure of reality and the way they view the rest of life. Life is not the same after such a shift as this. Some people may begin to look for someone to blame. But who to blame? If people do not get angry at the healer, they usually get angry at God for all the change, all the apparent chaos, all the feelings, all the transformation that healing brings. In the confusion which can accompany transformation what the client reports about the energy being channeled may even seem to be an invalidation of the healer or the healing process.

Sometimes, apparent resistance on the part of the client is not simply resistance. An "unsuccessful healing" is not necessarily unsuccessful. The truth is that a healer can never be sure of the part he or she plays in the karmic pattern of the client. A theory from physics which is applicable to this metaphysical process is *Heisenberg's uncertainty principle.*[72] Often the healer cannot fully comprehend the nature of the healing process because he or she is a part of that process. Every healer's intent is to heal. When a healing does not take place,

[72] See Rupert Sheldrake, *A New Science of Life: The Hypothesis of Formative Causation*, Los Angeles, California: J.P. Tarcher, 1981. See also Gary Zukav, *The Dancing Wu Li Masters*, New York: Bantam Books, 1980. This principle, which is the foundation of quantum mechanics, was formulated by the German physicist Werner Heisenberg (1901-1976) and won him the Nobel Prize in 1932. In essence the uncertainty principle states that "in the subatomic realm, we cannot know both the position and the momentum of a particle with absolute precision. We can know both, approximately, but the more we know about one, the less we know about the other..." Furthermore, all attempts to observe the electron alter the electron. In other words, the primary significance of the uncertainty principle is that we cannot observe something without changing it. What all this suggests is that "there exists an ambiguity barrier beyond which we can never pass without venturing into the realm of uncertainty. For this reason, Heisenberg's discovery became known as the 'uncertainty principle'." (Zukav, pp. 27, 111 and 112) Heisenberg's work greatly influenced the development of atomic and nuclear physics. Zukav's book, an overview of the "new physics", is written in beautifully clear language—with not a single mathematical equation—and illuminates the similarities between Eastern philosophies and physics (quantum mechanics).

sometimes this is not a reflection on either the client's resistance or the healer's ability. The apparent failure may not be a failure at all, but rather reflect the existence of a Greater Plan. Some people call this *karma*.[73]

Karma and Healing

Karma has been defined as many things. As a philosophical movement, metaphysical thought must be careful not to propagate a stagnant or punitive position on karma. The idea that an individual creates his illness often leads the ill person into feelings of guilt and powerlessness which result in further energy loss. If such feelings persist, the illness is likely to persist as well.

More than any other definition, my personal preference is to think of karma as a chosen learning process. A healer provides an opportunity for learning and change to take place in the life of the client. Such transformation might be considered payment for karmic debt. If a healer has a "karmic responsibility", it is to quicken the learning process, to teach the body to be more energy efficient and to model other ways of being. It is actually this learning process that allows energy to move freely and more efficiently in the body. When this occurs, one is most certainly more clearly connected to his higher destiny.

Definition of Health

At present, health in our country is defined as lack of disease. That is really not a reasonable definition for health. Health means "full of light". Less than "full of light"

[73] A more complete discussion of the concept of *karma* (or *karman*) will be found in Volume Two.

might be termed "disease". However, if we do not have an instrument to measure "full of light", we are left with the model of "normal health" that is deficient in many respects. The fact of the matter is we really have no concept of what "normal" is for the body. Therefore, it might behoove us all to change our view of health to include much broader terms.

As we explore the chakras one by one, we will begin to see that a healthy system implies much more than freedom from disease: vitality, appropriate feelings, appropriate thought process, a willingness to embrace change in our lives, creative self-expression and responsibility, intuitive understanding and a healthy spiritual relationship with the Ultimate Creative Force are all essential if we are to be "full of light" and full of life and well being.

MEDITATION ON THE CHAKRAS

One of the most ancient Yogic teachings about chakras is that they open when we inhale and close when we exhale. That is not quite true. What is implied is if we breathe deeply, we have more access to prana[74] energy or to chi (ki) energy (vital life force) than if we breathe shallowly.

To demonstrate, take a deep breath. Hold it. Exhale. Then immediately inhale quickly. And hold it. Exhale. Inhale again. Hold it. Exhale. Then just breathe normally if you can. If you feel more comfortable with your eyes closed, close them gently.

Next, imagine an energy that comes from the earth itself and enters your body through your feet. As energy starts to flow into you from the ground, notice whether you can feel it more in one foot than the other. Then begin bringing energy past your knees and into the core of your body.

As energy begins to enter the trunk of your body and to move up your spine, visualize red being in the area of the first center. You might take an extra breath to ensure that image, and then let the breath out.

Then as you inhale again, move to the second center. Envision orange in that second center. Exhale.

Inhale, moving up to the third chakra, visualize yellow there, and exhale.

Inhale, moving up to the heart chakra, envisioning green, and exhale.

Inhale, moving up to your throat, visualize blue, and exhale.

Continue the breathing as you move up to the third eye, visualizing a beautiful violet. Exhale.

Once more inhale, and, becoming

[74]   Prana is the Hindu, and chi or ki is the Oriental name for the vital life force or energy in the body, accessible through breath. Prana functions in conjuction with mind, in Hindu, manas. Pranayamas is the Yogic discipline dedicated to regulation of the breath and thus accessing vital energy. See Part Two for further discussion.

aware of the top of your head, visualize white light around your body, and exhale. Become aware again of your first chakra and the red color that is there. Visualize it as a plasmic energy field of red into which you can see. Look into that color and notice if there is an element in that light. Do you associate any gemstone with that red light? What kind of animal form do you associate with that color? Notice the actual color of the animal. Is it red or is it surrounded by red?

Now ask yourself if there are any people in your life now, or have there ever been, that spontaneously come into focus in this first center. Just make a mental note of it.

Then take a deep breath, visualize white light all around you again, and exhale.

Next, focus on your second chakra and the orange light that exists there. Looking into that field, see what element you associate with that orange light. Look for a gemstone that you associate with this frequency. Then, as you look through it, notice if there is an animal form that you see in this light. Notice what kind of animal and what color the animal actually is; is it orange or surrounded by orange? Look for any people that you know now, have known or will know who spontaneously come into this center.

Make a mental note of this world and take a deep breath. Surround yourself with white light again and then let go of the breath.

Move your awareness to your third center and see the yellow light that emanates from there. Look into this field of light. What elements do you associate with it? See if there is a gemstone that you also associate with this center. What kind of animal form appears here? What color is the animal if it is not yellow? Then see what people you spontaneously associate with this center.

Inhale deeply again. Surround yourself with white light. Exhale and relax.

Focus on your heart and your heart center, and look deeply into the beautiful green light that is there. Do you associate an animal with that center? Is there a gemstone that relates to your heart center? What people do you spontaneously recognize when you look into your own heart chakra?

Take another breath. Surround yourself with white light. Exhale and relax.

Now move up into your throat center, and visualize a beautiful blue light emanating from it. Looking deeply into the light, what element do you associate with this center? What gemstone do you associate with this center? What animal do you visualize here? Are there any people in your life now or in your past that you associate with this center? Make a note of what you found there.

Take a deep breath again. Surround yourself with white light, exhale and relax.

Focus now on the third eye, the sixth center. Notice the violet light that emanates from it. Look deeply into the light and envision whatever element you associate with this center. Is there a stone that appears here? What animal, if any, do you connect to this center? Are there any people that spontaneously come to mind when you focus on this chakra?

Take another deep breath. Surround yourself with white light, exhale and relax.

Focus on the crown center now and see the white light that radiates from it. Look deeply into the white light. See what elements you associate with it. Is there a stone that you visualize with this light? Is there an animal that appears here in the white light? When you look deeply into the white light, what people spontaneously appear to you? Make note of what you have seen.

Take a final deep breath. Circle yourself with white light, exhale and relax. As you relax, let go of any tension that you have, leaving it in the white light. Let your hands awaken. Let your feet awaken. Begin to bring energy back down your spine. Focus your awareness in the room. Open your eyes.

In this exercise if you did not visualize the traditional elements or animals in each chakra, do not be concerned. If, for instance, you visualized a horse instead of a snake in the first chakra, it does not matter. The purpose of this meditative exercise and of others throughout the book is to direct us toward our own internal place of silence where we, like the Rainbow Warrior, can begin to become aware of the chakras and of their subtle energies. Once we have achieved this kind of awareness, then these energy centers may become positive and effective dynamic forces within our lives and consciousnesses.

PART TWO

THE
FIRST
CHAKRA

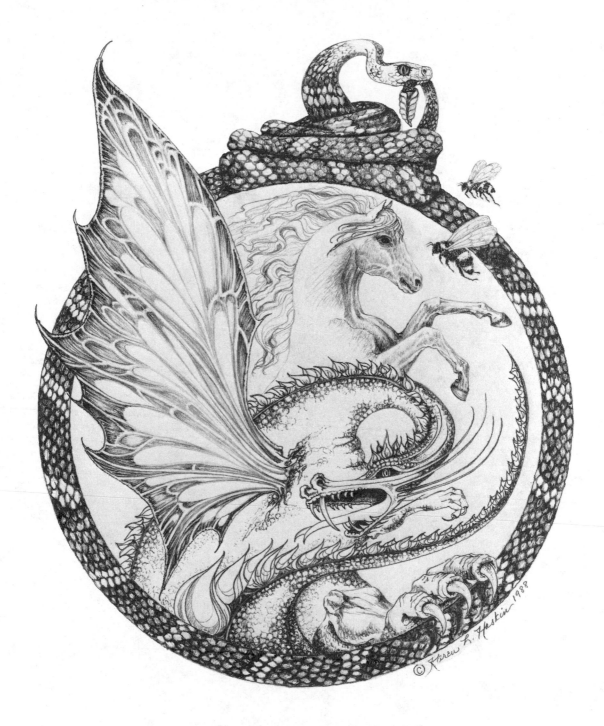

Fig. 1.1. ASSOCIATIVE ANIMALS OF THE FIRST CHAKRA
Illustration by Karen Haskin.

Chapter One

BEING ALIVE

The First Chakra: Our Life Force

Although the first chakra seems to be essential to the sustaining of life, here in the body, in the physical world, very little of value or authority has been written about it. The description given by Annie Besant in *Talks On the Path to Occultism* is representative of most of the modern literature on the subject:

> Kundalini...commonly lies sleeping in the chakra or force-centre at the base of the spine. If it is awakened prematurely, that is, before the man has purified his character of every taint of sensual impurity and selfishness, it may rush downwards and vivify certain lower centers in the body (used only in some objectionable forms of black magic), and irresistibly carry the unfortunate man into a life of indescribable horror; at best, it will intensify all that the man has in him, including such qualities as ambition and pride...[75]

From descriptions such as this, then, we would conclude that the importance of the

[75] Annie Besant and Reverend Charles W. Leadbeater, *Talks on the Path to Occultism*, Madras, India: Theosophical Publishing House, 1926, p. 405.

first chakra is that the "kundalini" is located there and that the best thing we can do is get the kundalini *out* of the first chakra as soon as possible since, if we leave it there, it will cause "indescribable horror"—and children.

Kundalini Energy: Keeping Us Alive

Not only is the kundalini located in the first chakra, but the first chakra is itself very often called the *kundalini*, which in Sanskrit means "serpent" or "sleeping snake".[76] The energies of this first center, our power, our sexuality, our "fire", are thus all connected to this serpentine image and its associations.

The energy of the first chakra is concentrated between the base of the spine and the pubic bone. This first center, however, encompasses the entire pelvic area of the body, including the genitals and the reproductive organs. Curiously, any material that has been written or collected about the chakras tends to have two or three sentences about sexuality in the first chakra and nothing more. It is as though sexuality were not one of the major and contributing forces in our lives, as though all of our emotional upset over mating had no effect on our spiritual lives at all. In fact, healers spend an extraordinary amount of time counseling people about their love lives and how their love lives affect their health and spiritual growth. Furthermore, anything that we investigate about the first chakra has to include how each individual's first chakra encounters other first chakras in the world, whether that encounter is intended or not.

The first chakra, like all of the chakras, has its own viewpoint, its own personality, if you will. It is athletic; it cares

[76] Edward Rice, *Eastern Definitions*, New York: Doubleday & Company, Inc., 1980, p. 231.

about contact. It cares about survival and sensuality, pleasure and power. It cares about proving whether or not we are alive, and it does not care how it goes about doing this. Being and staying alive is its prime objective.

Traditional Aspects of the First Chakra

Astrological Sign, Physical Element and Gemstone

Since the energy of the first chakra encompasses the pelvic area of the body, the astrological sign associated with the first chakra is often Scorpio because Scorpio rules the genitals. This is not to imply that all Scorpios are necessarily "first chakra people", only that the sign itself is associated with this first energy center whose main function is the creation and maintenance of life.

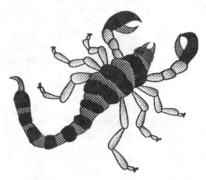

The element that is usually associated with the first chakra is fire, because of the heat experienced in the sensation mystically called the "rising of the kundalini". When people have this mystical opening, they generally experience a feeling of heat that starts at the base of the spine and burns its way to the top of the head.[77]

Fig. 1.2. SCORPIO. Because it rules the generative organs, the astrological sign of the scorpion is associated with the first chakra. Computer drawing by M.M. Smith/Techni-Visions.

Although most ancient texts associate the first chakra and the physical body with fire, alchemical texts usually designate the physical body with the element of earth. However, the "red dirt" or "clay" out of which mankind was created may, in fact, signify creation of the physical body out of fire: kabbalistically, Adam, or the Adamic man, is related to the Yod, or fire flame, which is the

[77] Cf. Chapter Two for further discussion of kundalini awakening.

117

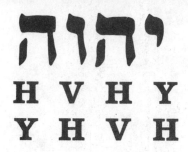

HVHY
YHVH

Fig. 1.3. THE TETRAGRAMMATON. In Hebraic tradition, the sacred Name of God is written as four letters (and read from right to left). The English equivalents are rendered YHVH and the name has come to be pronounced as Yahweh or, more incorrectly, Jehovah, although the ancient Hebrews recognized that there could be no name for the transcendent, unknowable aspect of God or Beingness. The first letter of the Tetragrammaton is Yod, symbolic of the Flame, the Cause, the One on which all things are based. It is the prototypical male principle. The second letter, He, is the female principle. Of the union of these two are begotten the Vau, the "Son" and the final He, called the "Daughter".

first letter of the sacred name of Jehovah (YHVH).[78]

It was generally believed in ancient civilizations that gemstones and the "noble" metals reflected or embodied certain powerful energies which might have a healing or strengthening influence on the wearer; or that these energies might assist the wearer in becoming attuned to certain inner energies, the energies of the various chakra centers.[79] Both the ruby and the fire opal are stones classically associated with the first chakra. Presumably, there is an opal for every chakra because opals exist in all the colors. Because of its association with surgery, the fire topaz is also connected with the first chakra which "rules" surgery. The ability to cut through flesh is related to the ability to remake it. This regenerative capacity is an essential function of the first chakra.

The Bee, the Dragon, the Horse and the Serpent

Throughout the ancient world, and even in more modern times, various animals, both historical and mythological, have been associated with the first chakra. Prominent among them are the bumblebee and the dragon. In the Western world, the horse is symbolic of the first chakra; and the snake, as suggested by the meaning of "kundalini", is most especially associated with the first chakra.

The image of the bumblebee is found in Crete and Egypt. In Crete the queen bee symbolized the mother goddess who created everything, nurtured everything and was the reason for being (see Fig. 1.5). In Egypt, the bumblebee was the sign of the female

[78] See S.L. MacGregor-Mathers,*The Kabbalah Unveiled,* New York, 1912. One of the best available texts which treats this essentially oral Jewish mystical tradition is A.E. Waite's *The Holy Kabbalah,* New Jersey: Citadel Press, n.d.

[79] See Raoul Birnbaum,*The Healing Buddha,* Boulder, Colorado: Shambhala Publications, Inc., 1979, p. 81. This author further cites several books, "of varying scholarly reliability" which treat this subject: G.F. Kunz, *The Curious Lore of Precious Stones,* New York: 1971 (original edition, 1913); B. Bhattacchayya, *Gem Therapy,* Calcutta: 1958; and W. T. Fernie, *The Occult and Curative Powers of Precious Stones,* Blauvelt, New York: 1973 (original edition, 1907).

pharaoh, the southern part of Egypt or the Upper Nile.[80]

The bee and other insects that move like the bee have a rhythmic movement in their legs and in their antennae. This movement relates to the first center. When that movement becomes exaggerated and accelerated, it is then associated with flight. In people when internal movement (or energetic vibration) becomes rapid, it can be said that we are "flying". We are lifting and moving, expanding and growing in a way that we had not before. Because of this association, the sound of buzzing is often related to the opening of the kundalini.[81] Consequently, the bumblebee became symbolic of the first chakra in the ancient world.

If we look at the symbology of the North and South American continents, crawlers and insects—worms, spiders, and lizards—are also associated with this center. In more ancient tradition, dragons are representative of this chakra. While the dragon has become a symbol of evil and sin to

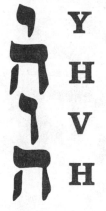

Fig. 1.4. By placing the four letters of the Tetragrammaton in a vertical column, a figure resembling a human form is produced. The Yod forms the head, the first He the arms and shoulders, the Vau the trunk of the body and the last He the hips and legs. Even if the Hebrew letters are exchanged for their English equivalents the form is not dramatically altered. (Hall, The Secret Teachings of All Ages, op. cit., p. CXXIV.)

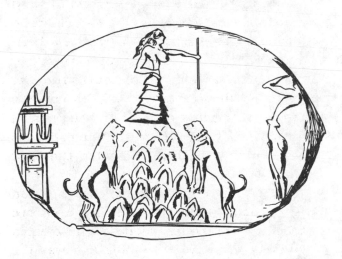

Fig. 1.5. THE GODDESS OF THE WORLD MOUNTAIN. Cretan sealing ca. 1500 B.C. Palace of Knossos. Note the similarity between the mountain and a beehive.

[80] See Joseph Campbell, The Masks of God: Occidental Mythology, New York: Penguin Books, 1978, pp. 50 - 51.

[81] See Motoyama, Theories of the Chakras, op. cit., p. 28; and Hall, Man: Grand Symbol of the Mysteries, op. cit., p. 214.

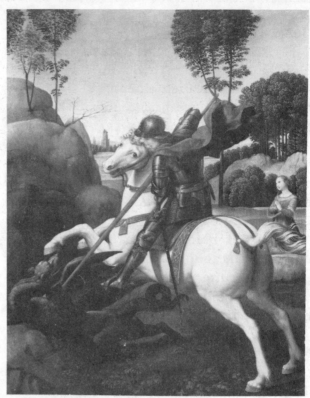

Fig. 1.6. ST. GEORGE AND THE DRAGON, Raphael. Courtesy National Gallery of Art, Washington, D.C.

Fig. 1.7. CADMUS FIGHTING THE DRAGON. Ancient Laconian cup. Courtesy of the Louvre.

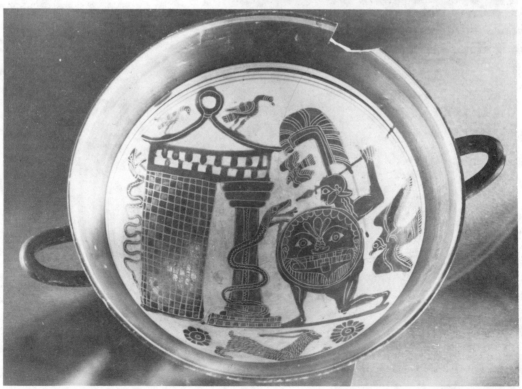

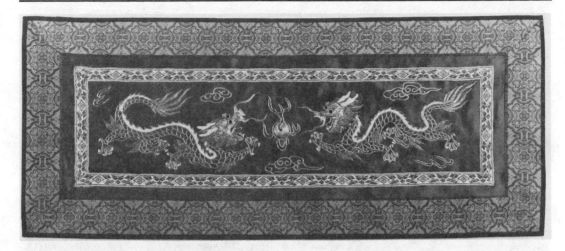

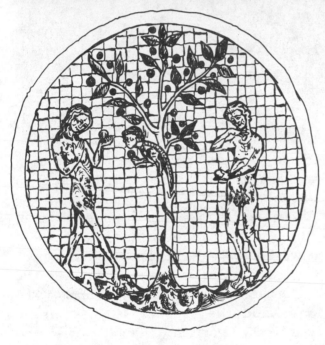

Fig. 1.8. THE IMPERIAL DRAGON. The dragon's prestige and beneficent nature were retained in Chinese culture where from ancient times it was the emblem of the Imperial family. Photo by Robert E. Williams/ Techni-Visions.

Fig. 1.9. MENORAH. England, 13th Century. A richly illustrated Menorah pictures the temptation of Adam and Eve by a cherubic looking serpent.

Christians, it represented just the opposite to many pre-Christian cultures. Throughout antiquity, "dragons" were held to be symbols of wisdom and immortality, of secret knowledge and of eternity. Adepts of Egypt, Babylon and India often referred to themselves as "Sons of the Dragon" and "Serpents" or "Sons of the Serpent God" during the presentation of the Mysteries.[82]

82 Blavatsky, op. cit., Vol. 1, pp. 379-380. In this section on the "Origin of the Satanic Myth", Blavatsky further comments that within these Mysteries, the initiate, himself a candidate for adeptship, would experience "terrible struggles...between himself and his (by magic) personified human passions, when the inner enlightened man had to either slay them or fail. In the former case, he became the 'Dragon-Slayer' as having happily overcome all the temptations; and a 'Son of the Serpent' and a Serpent himself, having cast off his old skin and being born in a *new* body, becoming a Son of Wisdom and Immortality in Eternity." (p. 380)

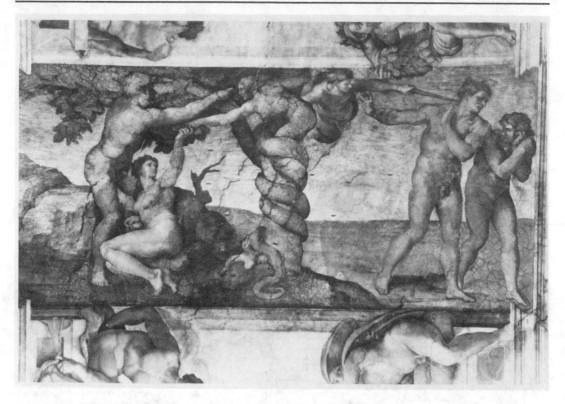

Fig. 1.10. THE FALL AND EXPUL-SION FROM EDEN. Michelangelo. Ceiling painting, Sistine Chapel, Vatican. Courtesy of the Vatican Museums.

The dragon's prestige and beneficent nature were retained in Chinese culture where from ancient times it was the emblem of the Imperial family as well as being symbolic of yang, the positive (+) principle of heaven, activity and maleness in Chinese cosmology.[83]

The horse and most especially the serpent are other first chakra animals. The horse and the serpent both originate symbolically in ancient tradition. Those who have studied Jungian symbology will find many sexual references to riding the horse;[84] but the association between sexuality and the horse dates back to the time of Alexander the Great and perhaps even further.

Jung left a wonderful legacy in psychotherapy regarding the disowned dark side of consciousness: the ever present promise that if we could identify and integrate our own disowned dark sides, inner as well as

[83] The *Encyclopaedia Britannica*, Vol. 4, 1985, p. 209. See Chapter Three of this section for a discussion of yin-yang.

[84] See Carl G. Jung, *Man and His Symbols*, New York: Doubleday & Company, Inc., 1964, and *Portable Jung*, ed. by Joseph Campbell, New York: Penguin, 1976.

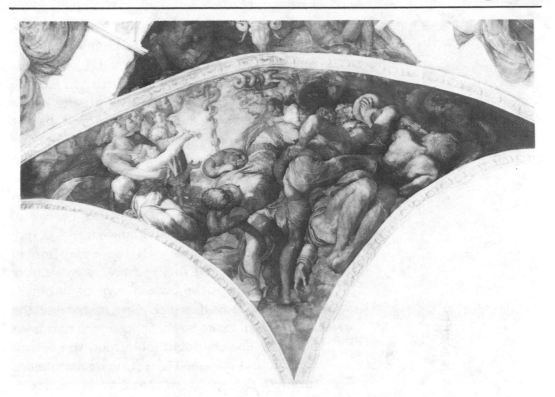

perhaps outer world peace would finally be possible. This is not an original idea. He came to that conclusion after studying esoteric lore.

The phallic symbolism of the horse and the power, sexuality and dark side of consciousness that are associated with the horse are all ideas which have also been associated with the image of the serpent in Freudian psychology. In the West, for nearly fifty years we have been inundated with the Freudian idea that snakes are phallic and in our dream life usually represent some deep, dark sexual desire. Consider this image next to that of the serpent of Eden who "seduced" Eve into disobedience, resulting in man's fall from grace and disfavor with God, and the snake appears to be a nasty fellow intent on causing us all kinds of misfortune; one, who in Annie Besant's words would carry us "into

Fig. 1.11. THE BRAZEN SERPENT OF MOSES. Michelangelo. Ceiling painting from the Sistine Chapel, Vatican. Courtesy of the Vatican Museums. "And the people spake against God, and against Moses, Wherefore have ye brought us up out of Egypt to die in the wilderness? for there is no bread, neither is there any water; and our soul loatheth this light bread. And the Lord sent firey serpents among the people, and they bit the people; and much people of Israel died. Therefore the people came to Moses, and said, We have sinned, for we have spoken against the Lord, and against thee; pray unto the Lord, that he take away the serpents from us. And Moses prayed for the people. And the Lord said unto Moses, Make thee a firey serpent, and set it upon a pole; and it shall come to pass, that everyone that is bitten, when he looketh upon it, shall live. And Moses made a serpent of brass, and put it upon a pole, and it came to pass, that if a serpent had bitten any man, when he beheld the serpent of brass, he lived. (Numbers 21:5-9)

a life of indescribable horror." However, since antiquity, the serpent, in its ability to slough its skin and thereby renew itself, has become a symbol of the mystery of rebirth. In fact the serpent who spoke to Eve was a deity in his own right, who had been honored in the Levant for seven thousand years before the composition of the Book of Genesis.[85] Within the ancient world, the serpent (like its larger cousin, the dragon) had long been representative of the adept, of his powers of immortality and "divine" knowledge.[86] Every culture of antiquity with the exception of Christians revered this symbol. Christianity elected to forget the brazen serpent of Moses (Numbers 21:5-9), which God instructed the Patriarch to make so that those who had been bitten by snakes might look upon the bronze serpent and live (see Fig. 1.11). Jesus himself implied the great wisdom and prudence symbolized by the serpent when he said, "Be ye wise as serpents and harmless as doves." (Matthew 10:16)[87] In fact throughout archaic literature, the usual mythological association of the serpent is not with deceit and corruption, as in Genesis, but with physical and spiritual well being and enlightenment.[88]

Snake Mythology: The Goddess Religion and the Power of the Undulate

Because the snake is so much a part of the first chakra and kundalini power, it is important that we take a closer look at its mythology and at some ancient practices surrounding it. Every ancient mythology at some point mentions that early in the evolutionary pattern of the world God (whatever god, goddess it is) creates

[85] Campbell, *The Masks of God: Occidental Mythology*, op. cit. This book, together with the remainder of Campbell's series: *The Masks of God: Primitive Mythology*, *The Masks of God: Oriental Mythology*, and *The Masks of God: Creative Mythology*, is a remarkable work of scholarship which examines world mythologies in the light of contemporary discoveries in archaeology, anthropology and psychology.

[86] Blavatsky, *The Secret Doctrine*, op. cit., Vol. II, p. 364.

[87] Ibid.

[88] See Joseph Campbell, *The Mythic Image*, Princeton, New Jersey: Princeton University Press, 1974, Chapter IV:2 "The Serpent Guide".

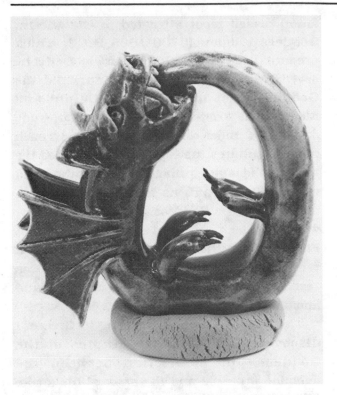

Fig. 1.12. DRAGON SWALLOWING TAIL. Throughout mythology the serpent has been viewed not only as a masculine but also as a feminine symbol. In this ceramic, the dual image of the snake as both male and female is suggested. Courtesy of Patricia Tawada. Photo by Robert E. Williams/Techni-Visions.

serpents.[89] While in our own culture (mainly as a result of Freudian influence) the snake has become associated with the masculine and male sexuality, I personally have never been impressed with the phallic symbolism of the serpent. Perhaps that is one reason I was led to explore the image of the snake as it appears in cultures other than our own. I discovered that mythically the serpent has been both masculine and feminine. In its essential nature as one which dwells both within waters and marshes and upon the earth, hanging from the branches of trees, the dual image of the serpent as both male and female is suggested. The phallic image is at once obvious; and, when the serpent is viewed as swallower, the female organ is also implied[90] (see Fig. 1.12).

As I further investigated the various religious cultures and their mythologies, I

[89] In Babylonia, it is the primeval waters of Tiamat which gives birth to serpents; the Persian *Bundahish* ("The Book of Creation") credits Angra Mainyu, the darker of the Dual Creators, with the creation of serpents, scorpions, frogs and lizards; in Greek myth, Gaea, mother earth, gives birth to the giant serpent, Typhon; in Chinese myth, the Dragon (which may be considered a serpent) is one of four animals who assist P'an Ku, in the actual creation of the world; and it is a giant serpent which lay at the roots of the World Tree, Yggdrasil, the sustaining force of the universe in Norse myth.

[90] Campbell, *The Masks of God: Occidental Mythology*, op. cit., p. 10 and p. 43.

found myself most attracted to the ancient Goddess religion (5700-1500 B.C.), which predates the religion of the male Deity by several thousand years. Not only did the Goddess exist in Egypt and Delphi and Eleusis; she existed throughout a multitude of cultures under different names.[91] In each of these cultures the Goddess represented the universal feminine principle of generation and regeneration. And, as a regenerative principle, it was the Goddess, not the male Deity, who first represented resurrection. Furthermore, the ancient Goddess religion revered the snake above all images, as it was seen to represent the feminine principle and feminine power.

When I was first traveling in Greece, I discovered, through my studies of the Goddess, the connection between the feminine principle and the snake: the snake is the power of the undulate, (i.e. vibration) and that is a feminine power. In addition to its undulating movement, the serpent's association with transformation and transmutable qualities—that which changes, sheds its skin and becomes new again—relates it more closely to the feminine. This transformative quality can be seen as more clearly feminine than masculine as it suggests the woman's monthly physiological cycle of "shedding" and "renewal" during menses.

The birthplace of the Goddess religion was Egypt. From there the Mysteries of Isis passed into Greek culture in the Orphic Mysteries at Delphi and the Mystery of Demeter (Ceres), the Universal Earth-Mother and her daughter, Persephone (Kore, the Universal Virgin-Mother)[92] at Eleusis. In *Book XI* of *The Golden Ass*, Lucius Apuleius, himself an initiate of Isis (c. 150 A.D.),

[91] For more information on the goddess religion, its practice, symbolism and historical significance, refer to Robert Graves, *The White Goddess*, New York: Vintage Books, 1959; John Blofield, *Bodhisattva of Compassion: The Mystical Tradition of Kuan Yin*, Lansing, Michigan: Shambhala Publications, 1978. Raphael Patai, *The Hebrew Goddess*, New York: Avon Books, 1978; Merlin Stone, *When God Was a Woman*, New York: Harcourt, Brace, Jovanovich; and *Ancient Mirrors of Womanhood*, Vols. I and II, New York: New Sibylline Books, 1979; Geraldine Thorstein, *God Herself*, New York: Doubleday & Company, Inc., 1980; Ann Belford Ulanov, *The Feminine*, Evanston, Illinois: Northwestern University Press, 1971; finally, see Campbell, *The Masks of God: Occidental Mythology*, op. cit., Chapters 1 and 2.

[92] According to mythology, the maiden Persephone conceived her son, Dionysus, by her father, Zeus. While she sat weaving in front of a cave where she had been left by her mother, Demeter, there guarded by the two serpents normally harnessed to Demeter's chariot, the young maiden was approached by her father, Zeus, who himself had taken the form of an immense snake. The virgin conceived of Zeus a son, Dionysus, the ever-living, ever-dying god of bread and wine, who was born and nurtured in that cave, torn to death there as a baby by the Titans sent by a jealous Hera, and resurrected through the intercession of the goddess Athene, who saved his heart and presented it to Zeus. According to one version of the myth, Zeus then accomplished the resurrection of Dionysus himself by swallowing his son's heart and giving birth to Dionysus once more. (Campbell, *The Masks of God: Primitive Mythology*, op. cit., p. 101.)

Fig. 1.13. THE GODDESS ISIS.
Drawing on papyrus from relief on a door of the third gilt shrine, tomb
of Tutankhamen, Valley of the Kings, 18th Dynasty. Cairo Museum.
Photo by Robert E. Williams/Techni-Visions.

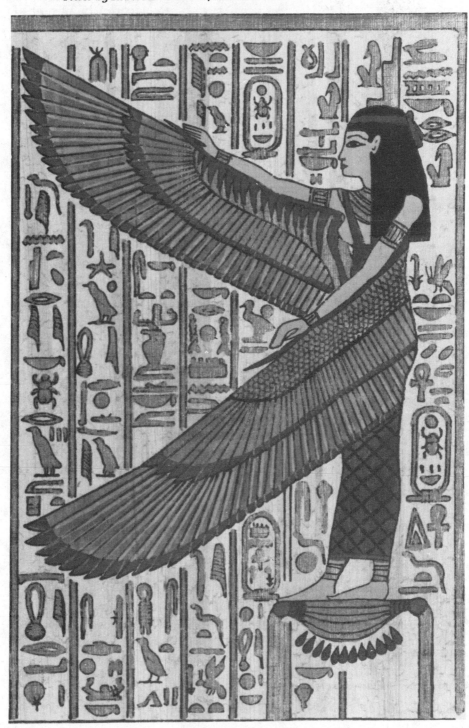

ascribes to the Goddess the following statement and attributes:

> I, who am Nature, the parent of things, the queen of all the elements, the primordial progeny of ages, the supreme of Divinities, the sovereign of the spirits of the dead, the first of the celestials and the uni-form resemblance of Gods and Goddesses. I who rule by my nod the luminous summits of the heavens, the salubrious breezes of the sea, and the deplorable silences of the realms beneath, and whose one divinity the whole orb of the earth venerates under a manifold form, by different rites and a variety of appellations. Hence the primogenial Phrygians call me Pessinunctica, the mother of the Gods; the Attic Aborigines, Cecropian Minerva; the floating Cyprians, Paphian Venus; the arrow-bearing Cretans, Diana Dictynna; the three-tongued Sicilians, Stygian Proserpine; and the Eleusinians, the ancient Goddess, Ceres. Some also call me Juno, others Bellona, others Hecate, and others Rhamnusia. And those who are illuminated by the incipient rays of that divinity, the Sun, when he rises...the Ethiopians, the Arii, and the Egyptians skilled in ancient learning, worshipping me by ceremonies perfectly appropriate, call me by my true name, Queen Isis.[93]

93 Hall, *The Secret Teachings of All Ages*, op. cit., p. XLV. For the original source, refer to Thomas Taylor, *Metamorphosis*, or *Golden Ass of Apuleius*, London, 1822 (cited in Hall, p. CCX). For another translation, refer to Campbell, *The Masks of God: Primitive Mythology*, op. cit., p. 56 (or see the original source, Apuleius, *The Golden Ass*, trans. W. Adlington, Book XI, as cited in Campbell). *The Golden Ass*, purported to be a novel of Lucius Apuleius, is almost definitely a thinly disguised revelation of an initiate's experience of the Mysteries of Isis.

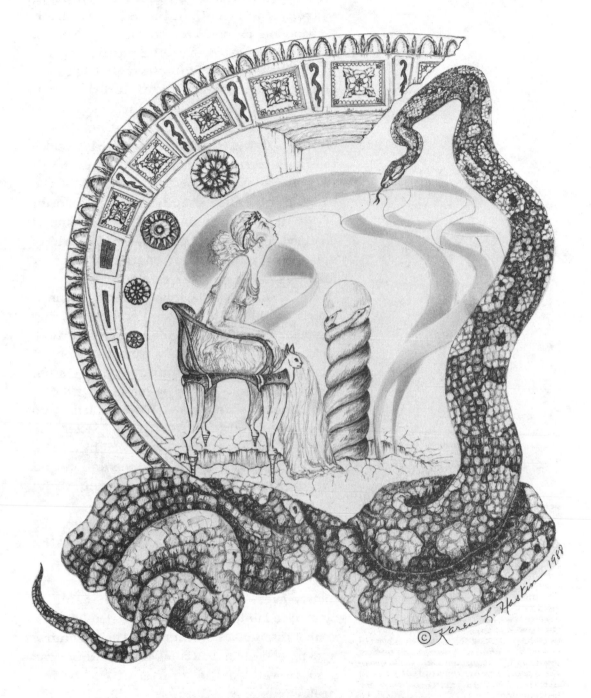

Fig. 1.14. THE ORACLE OF DELPHI
"Let no one without clean hands come near."
Illustration by Karen Haskin.

At Eleusis, Demeter's agonizing search for her abducted daughter, Persephone, parallels the sorrowful journey of Isis as she sought her brother-spouse, Osiris, in Egyptian legend. In both mythologies the efforts of the two goddesses to bring their missing relatives back from the realm of the dead are ultimately realized, although not entirely: Osiris, though resurrected, decides to remain in the realm of the dead; Persephone is returned to the land of the living, but because she has eaten of the fruit of the dead, one pomegranate seed, she is destined to return to the dark underworld of spirits for one-third of each year forever after.[94]

Like the similarity of the myth of Isis-Osiris to that of Demeter-Persephone, the Egyptian story of the dying-resurrected God, Osiris, differs only slightly from the story of Dionysus, its Greek counterpart.[95] Osiris, who was cut into pieces by his brother, Seth, was resurrected by his sister-wife, Isis, who found all of Osiris's bodily parts (except his phallus, which had been swallowed by a fish). She brought him to life by incantation and thereupon miraculously (immaculately) conceived of him, their son, Horus.

Because of its nature and form, the snake, then, was seen to symbolize the powers of generation and regeneration, and by association, to represent the Goddess. In nearly every culture the serpent came to symbolize life itself, which circulates (like the snake) through all of Nature.[96] The generative and regenerative power of the Goddess was also viewed as the source of the body's healing capacity. Because of this, both the snake and the Goddess it represented came to symbolize healing among the ancients.

Snakes did not take on phallic

[94] For a summary of the myth of Demeter and Persephone, refer to Campbell, *The Masks of God: Primitive Mythology*, op. cit., pp. 183-185.

[95] Cf. note 92 this chapter. Also see Campbell, *The Masks of God: Primitive Mythology*, op. cit., pp. 424-426 for the story of the murder, death and resurrection of Osiris. Upon comparison of the Isiac and the Eleusinian-Orphic Mysteries with that of Christianity in which the Virgin Mary conceives by God the Holy Ghost (in the form of a dove) God the Son, who is born in a cave, dies and is resurrected to be ever present in the bread and wine of the Mass, we are once more reminded that all religious mythologies are reflections of one common spiritual truth.

[96] Albert Pike, *Morals and Dogma of the Ancient and Accepted Scottish Rite of Freemasonry*, Charleston, West Virginia, 1921, Chapters XXIV and XXV.

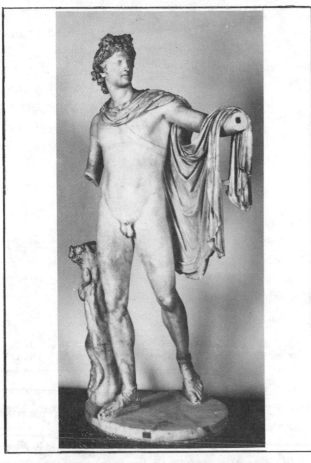

Fig. 1.15. APOLLO BELVEDERE. Carrera marble. Copy of a 4th c. statue. Original in the Vatican. Courtesy Vatican Museums.

[97] *Oracle* may be used to refer to the place of prophecy, to the prophet or to the prophecy itself.

[98] According to Schuré, it was Orpheus, the son of a priestess of Apollo and an initiate of the Egyptian Mysteries, who established the solar cult of Apollo at Delphi. After having experienced the Mysteries of Isis and Osiris, Orpheus returned to his native Thrace "bearing an initiation-name which he had acquired as a result of his ordeals, and had received from his teachers as a sign of his mission... Orpheus of Arpha, which means *the one who heals with light.*" (*The Great Initiates*, op. cit., p. 230.) For further discussion of Orpheus and his position in Greek history and myth, refer to Fabre d'Olivet, *Golden Verses of Pythagoras*, trans. Redfield, New York: Putnam & Sons, 1925 (cited in Schuré, op. cit., p. 515). It was in Thrace and at Delphi that Orpheus established the Mysteries of Dionysus, whose life, death, and resurrection mythologically corresponds exactly to that of Osiris of Egypt, Tammuz-Dumuzi of Babylonia, Adonis of Sumeria, Atys (Attis) of Phrygia, to that of Cashmala of the Cabiric Mysteries of Samothrace, of the Viking god, Odin, and of Jesus Christ in Christianity. (See Hall, *The Secret Teachings of All Ages*, op. cit., for further details of these corresponding mythologies.)

symbolism until the Temple of Apollo overtook the Temple of Delphi. Delphi was an *oracle*[97] that had always been controlled by women, and the woman, or head priestess, in charge was called the Pythoness. According to mythology, the original name of the oracle was Pythos, so called because its chambers were the home of the great serpent, Python, who had crept out of the slime left by the receding flood of Deucalion's time. Apollo climbed the side of Mount Parnassus, killed the serpent and threw its body down the fissure of the oracle. After the last Pythoness was slain, as religious power historically transferred from the hands of women into the hands of men, the Temple of Apollo was erected at Delphi.[98]

Figs. 1.16 and 1.17. OSIRIS AND DIONYSUS. The Egyptian story of the dying-resurrected god, Osiris, differs only slightly from the Greek myth of Dionysus. In both mythologies, the deity is murdered, torn to pieces and then resurrected through the intercession of a goddess. Isis, the sister-wife of Osiris, brings him to life by incantation and thereupon conceives of him, their son, Horus. The goddess Athene saves the heart of Dionysus and presents it to Zeus, who, according to one version of the myth, then accomplishes the resurrection of Dionysus himself by swallowing his son's heart and giving birth to Dionysus once more.

Fig. 1.16. TUT-ANKH-AMUN'S MUMMY dressed as Osiris.

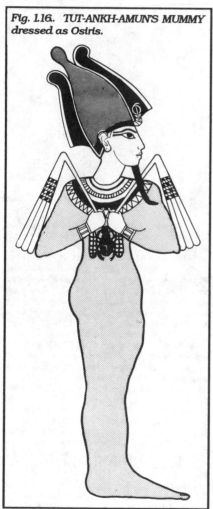

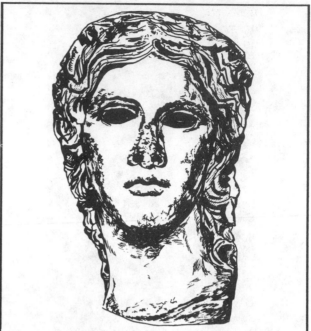

Fig. 1.17. HEAD OF THE YOUNG DIONYSUS. Late Hellenistic Carving. Found near Rome. British Museum.

From that time on the Sun God, surnamed the Pythian Apollo, gave oracles from the temple.

After being conquered by Apollo, it was said that the spirit of Python remained at Delphi as the representative of his conqueror. Virgin maidens, who were called the Pythiae and constituted that order now known as the Pythian priesthood, were allowed to remain to become the "voice" of the oracle; it was with the aid of the effluvium of Python that the priestess was able to gain rapport with the god.[99] The ancient initiate, Iamblichus, in his dissertation on *The Mysteries*, describes how the spirit of the oracle took control of the Pythoness and manifested through her:

> "...The prophetess in Delphi, whether she gives oracles to mankind through an attenuated and fiery spirit, bursting

99   Hall, *The Secret Teachings of All Ages*, op. cit., p. LXII.

from the mouth of the cavern; or whether being seated in the adytum on a brazen tripod, or on a stool with four feet, she becomes sacred to the God; whichsoever of these is the case, she entirely gives herself up to a divine spirit, and is illuminated with a ray of divine fire. And when, indeed, fire ascending from the mouth of the cavern circularly invests her in collected abundance, she becomes filled from it with a divine splendor. But when she places herself upon the seat of God, she becomes coadapted to his stable prophetic power: and from both of these preparatory operations she becomes wholly possessed by the God. And then, indeed, he is present with and illuminates her in a separate manner, and is different from the fire, the spirit, the proper seat, and, in short, from all the visible apparatus of the place, whether physical or sacred.[100]

Apollo, the sun god, then, took on the power of the snake, and the snake became his symbol. Thereafter male fertility became related to the serpent.

Ida and Pengali: Dual Male and Female Aspects of the First Chakra

The serpent then has both mythically and mystically come to represent several powers. In its connection to the Pythoness of Delphi, it is a symbol of prophecy; in its association with the Goddess, it represents

100 Ibid. For the original source, see Thomas Taylor, *Iamblichus on the Mysteries*, London, 1895. For a further description of the Pythoness of Delphi, refer to the *Encyclopaedia Britannica*, Vol.1, 1985, p. 484 and Vol. 8, pp. 974-975; Schuré, op. cit., Chapter 32, gives an initiate's observation of the oracle.

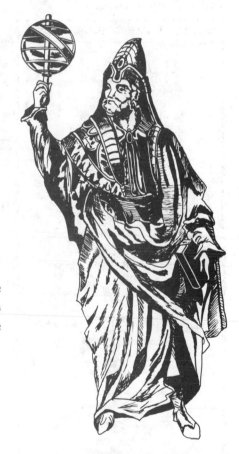

Fig. 1.18. HERMES TRISMEGISTUS. The "thrice-greatest" priest, philosopher and king of Greek and Medieval tradition was known as Thoth or Tehuty (Djhuty) to the ancient Egyptians. From Historia Deorum Fatidicorum.

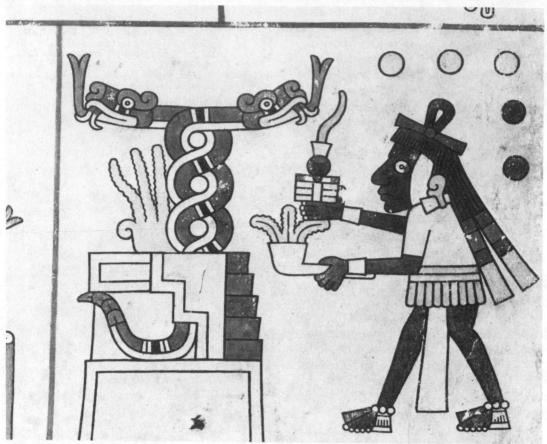

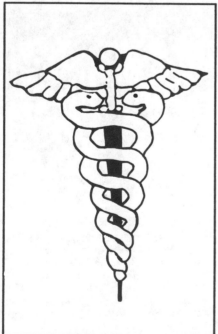

Fig. 1.19. ALTAR OF THE CADUCEUS. In America, as well as in the ancient cities of Egypt, Greece, Sumeria and India, the Serpent was seen to symbolize the power of resurrection over the physical death of the body. Above, a worshipper offers incense and gifts to a serpent deity in the form of a modified caduceus. From the Codex Fejervary Mayer, a 15th century Mixtec picture manuscript. Courtesy of National Museums and Galleries on Merseyside—Liverpool Museum.

Fig. 1.20. THE CADUCEUS. This symbol of the medical profession first appeared in antiquity as the staff of the legendary Egyptian High-priest, Tehuty, who is alleged to have brought to Egypt the "divine knowledge" of sacred healing. The caduceus itself unmistakenly resembles the image of the Ida and Pengali serpents who "rise" to the top of the spine in the mystical experience of the kundalini awakening.

the feminine powers of generation and regeneration; and through these aspects, it has come to symbolize healing. Even today, the caduceus, a staff around which two snakes are entwined, is recognized as the general emblem of the medical profession (see Fig. 1.20).

In antiquity, the caduceus first appears as the staff of the legendary Egyptian High Priest, Tehuty, later called Hermes (or Hermes Trismegistus) by the Greeks (see Fig. 1.18). Egyptian tradition maintains that this "Thrice-Greatest" priest, philosopher and king escaped the destruction of Atlantis, where he had been the premier Atlantean High Priest, and brought to Egypt the sacred and secret doctrine,[101] among which was the "divine knowledge" of sacred healing.

The caduceus also appears as the associative symbol of the later Greek physician Asklepios (Aesculapius in the Latinized form), who was probably a student and initiate of Tehuty, although in Greek mythology, Tehuty, Thoth, Hermes and Asklepios all share essentially the same personage. According to this myth, Asklepios was punished by Zeus for bringing a mortal back from the dead (again the theme of resurrection or regeneration). Eventually Asklepios and his two daughters, Panacea and Hygeia, established a healing temple which became the Oracle of Epidauros. Here both physical and psychic healing took place. One of the most famous cures was that attained by sleeping overnight within the temple. The sufferers not only benefited in sleep from the healing energies within the sacred precinct but would often be granted a dream-message or vision from God, which would serve to guide the patient toward future spiritual development. Perhaps because of this

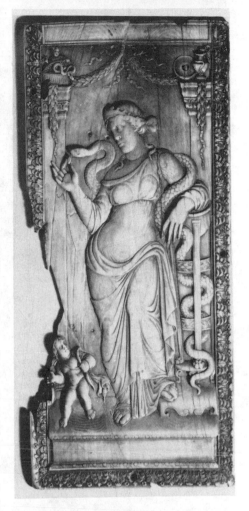

Fig. 1.21. HYGEIA. 4th. c. ivory diptych. Courtesy of National Museums and Galleries on Merseyside —Liverpool Museum.

101 See Hall, *The Secret Teachings of All Ages*, op. cit., pp. XXIV - XL.

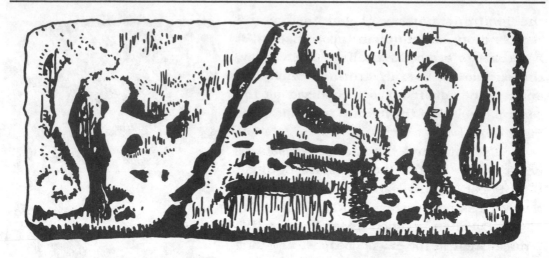

Fig. 1.22. DEITY WITH WOR-SHIPPERS AND SERPENTS ca. 2000 B.C. Indus Valley seal.

Fig. 1.23. LORD OF THE TREE OF TRUTH. ca. 2500 B.C. This extended drawing taken from an ornamented Sumerian ritual cup of the same period as the Indus Valley seal reveals the Mesopotamian serpent-god Ningishzida in his dual aspect as a pair of copulating vipers. Entwined about an axial rod, they suggest both the caduceus of Hermes-Thoth-Asklepios and the pictorial representation of the rising Serpent Power of awakened kundalini.

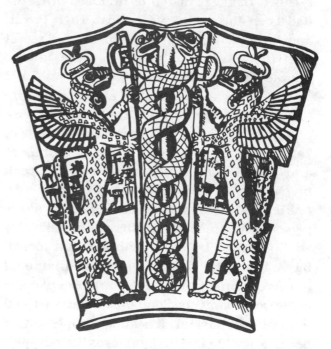

102 Joscelyn Godwin, *Mystery Religions in the Ancient World*, San Francisco, California: Harper & Row, Publishers, 1981, p. 44. Also see Jeannine Parvatti, *Hygieia: A Woman's Herbal*, Berkeley, California: Bookpeople, 1978, p. ix, and Campbell, *The Mythic Image*, op. cit., pp. 284-287.

Asklepios came to be regarded as one who healed not only sickness but the soul as well. As such the serpent acquired even further significance as symbolizing both the subtle "currents" of the body and the "spiral windings of the soul's evolutionary path".102

This duality is represented in Hindu myth and mysticism by the *Ida* and the *Pengali* (or *Pingala*). They are the female and male serpents respectively that intertwine in the body, the source of energy flow that moves from center to center up the spine. When these "snakes" have risen to the top of the spine in the rising kundalini experience, some people say they then sense an opposing downward force which is called *sushumna*. As sensation moves downward, one has an experience of complete awareness of all the chakras "awakening" and the energy flowing freely between them.[103] Pictorially, the caduceus can be seen to represent this awakening of the seven chakra centers by the rising Serpent Power of the kundalini (see Figs. 1.22 and 1.23).

Initiation and the First Chakra

Kundalini Initiation and the Siddhi Powers

Not only because of its association with the Oracle but because of its mystical connection to the rising and awakening of the kundalini, the serpent is also linked to abilities which have come to be known in the consciousness movement as "siddhi powers". In Hindu "siddhi" means "perfection", and the powers refer to those usually acquired through the mastery of the higher stages of yoga. Generally, ten or twelve siddhi powers are listed, depending upon the discipline studied. Clairvoyance, clairaudience, teleportation, telekinesis, precognition, levitation, telepathy, clairsentience, invisibility, bilocation, materialization and healing are some examples of these major powers.

The kundalini is the sleeping snake; according to Hindu tradition, it sits coiled

[103] For the source of these terms refer to the *Shri-Jabala Darshana*, the *Cudamini*, the *Yoga-Shikka* and the *Shandilya Upanishads*. A summary of the information found in these texts may be found in Motoyama, op. cit., Chapter V. In brief, the *sushumna* is a nerve canal which follows the spine. Although descriptions of its point of origin vary, it is generally agreed that it begins at the tip of the coccyx (the first chakra) and travels up the spinal cord to the top of the head (the Brahman Gate), through which prana (breath) and kundalini energy are said to enter and exist. In Chinese medicine, the governor vessel meridian seems to closely correspond to the *sushumna* (Motoyama, p. 141).

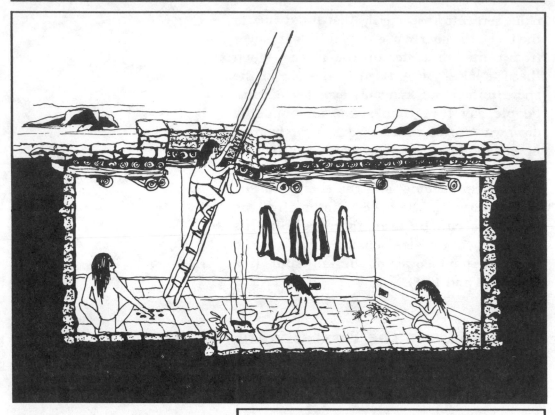

Fig. 1.24. A KIVA. Sectional view
showing interior and construction
details of a subterranean kiva.

Fig. 1.25. Top: HOPI KIVA. Floor plan
of one of the many Hopi-like kivas at
Awatovi. Bottom: Typical mural
fragment. The figure represented is
probably Ahola Katcina (kachina),
symbol of the coming of the sun.
Illustrations based on those by
Thomas E. Mails in The Pueblo
Children of the Earth Mother, © 1983
by Thomas E. Mails. Used by
permission of Doubleday, a division of
Bantam, Doubleday, Dell Publishing
Group, Inc.

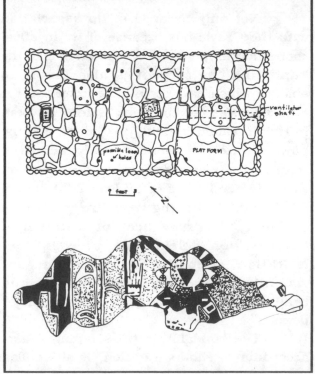

three and a half times at the base of the spine. When it is awakened, however, it rises (hopefully) to center around and stop near the pineal and pituitary glands, which sit very close together near the thalamus and the hypothalamus in the midbrain. When the Serpent Power becomes activated in this way there can be a wonderful experience of "seeing" without the presence of physical light. If we sit in darkness fully awake and conscious, we eventually begin to see, though there is no source of light, because the chemical reaction of the inner synapse of the body becomes visible. We begin to see and sense and feel, actually feeling as much as we are seeing. Here on our own continent many of us have gone through Native American kiva[104] initiations that duplicate this same process, where, in darkness, imagery comes forth from the inside. In the ancient world, a major purpose of initiation in all the mysteries was to awaken this sight. Theoretically, after one experiences the rising of the kundalini—the awakened Serpent Power—not only "sight" but all the siddhi powers are made available to the newly conscious initiate.

In the mythologies of China and India and in particular those of Greece and Egypt, the myth of the snake as part of this kundalini initiation process is predominant. Although the initiates into the ancient Mystery Religions were sworn to secrecy regarding their experiences, the few personal accounts which have survived[105] make it clear that the purpose of these initiations was the same in all cultures: the function of all Lesser Mysteries, or the lower grades of initiation, was to convey to the initiates information about the nature of the higher worlds, while the purpose of the Greater Mysteries, or the higher degrees of initiation,

[104] A *kiva* is a Pueblo Indian (mainly Hopi and Zuni) ceremonial structure. It is usually round and partly underground. Although its most important purpose is for ritual ceremonies such as the kundalini initiation, the *kiva* is also used for political meetings and less frequently, for social gatherings of the men of the village.

[105] Iamblichus (*De Mysteriis, V*), Plato (*Phaedrus*), Proclus (*In Republicam, I*), Plutarch (*Fragment 178* of Stobaeus) and Apuleius (*Metamorphosis, XI*), have all given some personal account of their experience of the Mysteries. Apuleius's account has been described as "one of the most persuasive descriptions of mystical experience to have survived from the ancient world." (Godwin, op. cit., p. 77) Although sworn to secrecy as an initiate himself, Apuleius used the persona of Lucius, his fictional hero, to reveal as much of the Isiac (Eleusinian) mysteries as his conscience would allow. With the exception of the thorough and rich descriptions of Schuré (*The Great Initiates*), whose sources are unidentified and Dudley Wright (*The Eleusinian Mysteries and Rites*, London: Theosophical Publishing House, n.d.), Apuleius's account is the most complete description of the ancient initiation that exists. For further reference and descriptions of the Mystery Religions and their initiations, see G.R.S. Mead, *Orpheus*, London, 1965, and *The Eleusinian and Bacchic Mysteries*, New York, 1891; R.G. Wasson, et al, *The Road to Eleusis: Unveiling the Secrets of the Mysteries*, New York: Harcourt, Brace, Jovanovich, 1978; as well as Godwin and Pike. The account of Apuleius may be found in both Godwin and Pike (Chapters XXIII and XXIV), the latter of whom supplies not only a history of the evolution of the initiations but also rich details of the preparation, the accouterments and the meaning of the different initiations within the various cultures.

139

was to bring the initiate into direct contact with the beings who inhabit these higher worlds. Although it has been suggested by some scholars[106] that the Mysteries were merely a sacred drama staged by actors to fill an impressionable audience with holy terror, the multi-pillared architecture of several of the temples precludes this; there simply was no room for a stage. Not only the temple structure but the personal accounts of ancient initiates indicate that something must have happened on the psychic plane which touched every person present.[107]

In the Native American tradition, as well as in Hinduism and Buddhism, that psychic plane, that inner "invisible" world from which, in darkness, imagery comes forth, is the "other world", or the real world; what we all see "normally" is the world of maya, the false world, the world that is not but appears to be. That difference becomes an important one in terms of discussing and understanding kundalini initiation.

Greece: Initiation in the Tholoi

While the Lesser Mysteries, the lower initiations, were conducted collectively, the Greater Mysteries were conducted individually. Many initiates into the Lesser Mysteries were never allowed admittance into the higher initiations. Those who were generally had to wait a specified period of time, usually from five to seven years or longer, before being permitted to participate. It took that long for the candidate to prepare, for the Greater Mysteries were intended to take him through the gates of death.

As in shamanic, Masonic and other later initiations, the

[106] *Encyclopaedia Britannica*, Vol. 24, 1985, pp. 703-709.

[107] Godwin, op. cit. p. 33.

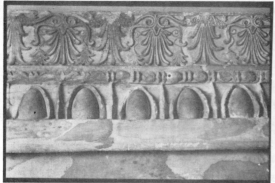
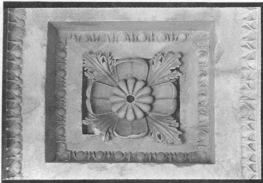

candidate was placed in a trance, his consciousness taken out of his body, and in this state he experienced higher states of being and met some of the denizens of the invisible worlds. Some were demonic, others beneficent... Through direct experience the candidate would learn that the gods he worshipped were perfectly real. Then he would return to earth fully convinced of his immortality and prepared to meet death fearlessly, knowing it as the gate to freedom and his soul's true home.[108]

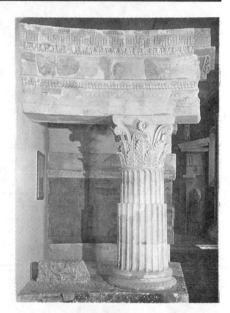

Figs. 1.26. EPIDAUROS. Top: detail of the temple walls. Note the egg-like image in the picture at above-left. The egg, like the serpent, was a symbol of the Goddess, as well as a representation of the entire universe. Bottom: the temple columns.

The kundalini initiation was a major part of these Greater Mysteries.

In Greece, the kundalini initiation in the Tholoi or Temple involved isolating an initiate in a subterranean maze. At Epidauros, there was a labyrinth under a rotunda, or ethilos, as it is called. The ethilos was a beautiful round chapel with lovely columns. An inner sanctuary existed under a keystone in the floor. An initiate would be dropped into the labyrinth through the hole made by the removal of the keystone (or capstone). Then the capstone would be replaced. Underground, there was a series of

108 Ibid, p. 35.

concentric passageways cut in such a way as to form a maze, and within that maze were snakes. The initiate was required to live in that underground maze for nine days in total darkness with no food or water—and to avoid the snakes. If the initiate survived, when he was brought out, he was to report what had occurred in and around the country while he was in the labyrinth. Thus, staying alive was only the first part of the test. Proper use of inner sight and psychic awareness was an additional part of the challenge.

There were similar initiations at Eleusis and at Delphi. Since the oracle at Delphi was originally dedicated to the Pythoness, its ethilos undoubtedly held pythons, and the initiate had to keep the pythons from squeezing him or her to death.

Fig. 1.27. THE GREAT PYRAMID OF CHIOPS. Initiation probably took place in both the King's and Queen's chambers. From Charles Piazzi Smythe, Life and Work at the Great Pyramid, Edinburgh: Edmonton & Douglas, 1867.

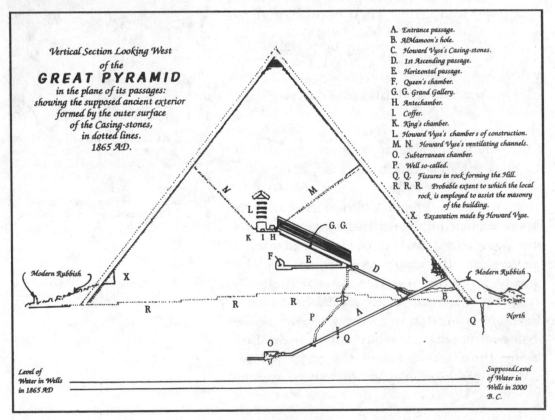

Egypt: Initiation in the Pyramids

The Egyptians also had a very interesting kundalini initiation.[109] Candidates
studied for about twenty-eight years before
they were sufficiently prepared to take it. The
initiates would ready themselves by a week of
dieting, fasting, praying and doing ablutions
in the Queen's Chamber of the large pyramid.
Then they were wrapped in linen as a
mummy, prayed over, carried by someone else
into the King's Chamber, and put into a
sarcophagus. A 2500 pound lid was placed
on the sarcophagus; the initiates would go
into a kind of suspended animation and leave
their bodies. While in this out-of-body state,
they traveled to the four corners of Egypt.
Nine days later, the initiates were removed
and unwrapped. If they were still alive, they
would receive the privilege of taking the final
test, which was to tell the presiding priest
(who had already been informed by four
runners who had come from the four corners
of Egypt) what had happened throughout the
country over those nine days.

The Eleusinian Mystery

Like the initiation within the pyramids,
there was a further test at Eleusis, but unlike
the pyramid initiation, it did not involve astral
projection. The mystery which occurred here
involved a beautiful metamorphosis.

Sadly, today the fields of Eleusis,
which are located between Athens and the
harbor-shipping port of Pereas, consist of no
fewer than a dozen factories and two auto
salvage yards. However, there is a strange

109 In addition to those references already
cited, see Hall, *The Secret Teachings of All
Ages*, p. XLI, for a further discussion of
initiation in the King's Chamber of the
Great Pyramid.

143

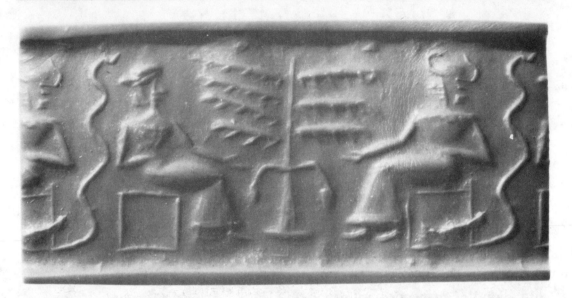

Fig. 1.28. THE GODDESS OF THE TREE OF LIFE ca. 2500 B.C. Sumeria. The female figure at left is most likely the goddess Gula-Bau, while the male on the right, who is a god, as evident from his horned lunar crown, is likely her son-spouse, Dumuzi, "Son of the Abyss, Lord of the Tree of Life", the ever-dying, ever reborn Sumerian prototype of the resurrected savior. Courtesy of the British Museum.

phenomenon attached to those fields. Parallel to the modern highway that connects Athens and Pereas is another road which leads to a sacred lake. This lake is exactly opposite the ocean, but it is not at sea level as it should be; it is seven feet higher than sea level. That is because it sits on a magnetic field.[110] This magnetic field marks the exact location of the sacred valley where the ancient Eleusinian Mystery Temple once stood.

The Temple of Eleusis was regarded as, in some sort, the common sanctuary of the whole earth, where religion had brought together all that was most imposing and most august.[111] Prospective initiates prepared themselves for seven years, and at the end of that seven year period they went to Eleusis. There they experienced the mystery of Demeter, whose name means "to measure". One had to measure up, as it were, to her standard, in order to pass the mystery. The mystery at Eleusis was in most ways similar to the mystery in the Epidauran and the Aesculapian mystery schools: one would go into a circular shrine or sanctuary and be

[110] This was my observation at the site.

[111] Pike, op. cit. p. 379.

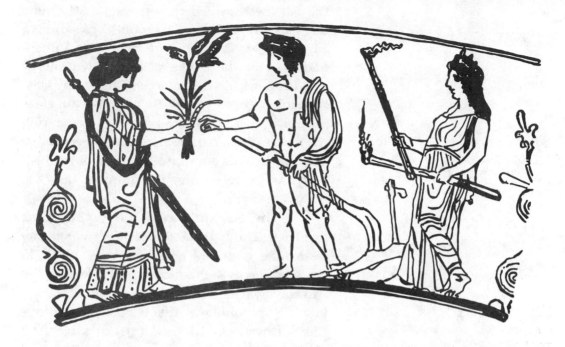

dropped down into a subterranean labyrinth, over which the capstone would be placed; the initiate remained in that labyrinth for nine days, in the dark, with snakes. At the end of those nine days, if the initiate were still alive and had not starved, he would be taken out. This, however, is where the similarity ends.

The Eleusinian initiate was sent in with seven kernels of wheat, each of which was to have been germinated into a stalk by the time he came out. There is only one way in which to accomplish this: if one could somehow manage to concentrate the energy of the Atman and the Brahman, the two highest chakra centers, between his hands, staying in prayer the entire nine days. Obviously one could not use his hands to defend himself against the serpents because he had to make enough light for those seeds to sprout. The initiate had to "measure up" as Demeter did, and what Demeter brought the world was grain. One had nine days to make grain in

Fig. 1.29. DEMETER, TRIPTOLEMUS AND PERSEPHONE. THE GREEK TRIAD. Demeter, at left, is handing grain to her fosterling, Triptolemus, who holds a "crooked plow". Persephone stands behind him, two torches in her hands denoting her queenship of the Underworld. From a red-figured cup discovered in the precincts of Eleusis.

the darkness, which corresponds to the nine days of the Goddess's moon cycle during which the earth becomes fertile. The initiate had to grow the stalks with his own energy and light, with the life force of his own body. He could never let go of the grain because the moisture to grow the stalks had to come from the sweat of his hands. He could never let go because he was growing the wheat in his own body, as Demeter grew the grain in her own body, the earth.

The Navajo have nearly the same mystery. The highest ceremonial Navajo way is to take grains of corn and grow them in one's hands in the darkness of the kiva in the eleven days of the recitation of the Navajo law.[112] The only way this is possible is if one has an awakened kundalini, an alive first chakra.

Modern Initiation

When we consider the power, the light, the surrender and the trust of these ancient initiations, our modern idea of initiation seems rather inferior by comparison. Among the ancients, certainly there was only a small group of people who ever took initiation.[113] In Egypt this was certainly true, and there was only a small number of Greeks that passed the Eleusinian mysteries as well. Likewise, only a small number of Jews went into the desert for forty days and forty nights, the amount of time required for the process of initiation in Hebraic tradition. In modern society there is a great lack of understanding of the kind of preparation necessary for initiation as well as of the transformation which initiation inevitably brings. This is especially true of kundalini initiation, which is intended to awaken our entire physical, as

---

[112] Navajo oral tradition.

[113] Words above the entrance to the temple at Eleusis which invited to approach only he who was "of clean hands and ingenuous speech, free from all pollution, and with a clear conscience" (Pike, op. cit. p. 357) and a similar warning above the temple entrance at Delphi ("Let no one without clean hands come near") served to dissuade many who gleaned from those words a warning of the great challenge which resided within.

well as spiritual consciousness. Despite this
lack of preparation, each of us goes through
initiation of some kind, with or without
realization of the experience.

Most "seekers" experience a similar
initiation process: some reality construct with
which they normally identify alters, and they
are taken into a state in which "the world" as
they know it is not the way it "should" be.
They are taken into a mystical state where
everything has shifted. Usually the first
experience of the world being other than how
they know it to be is really frightening.
However, the more often a seeker goes into an
alternate reality, the less frightening and
confusing it becomes. In order to understand
the meaning of modern kundalini initiation,
we need to further explore the first chakra,
kundalini power and the physical body.

Chapter Two

KUNDALINI: SEAT OF THE PHYSICAL BODY

The Root Chakra

In the ancient Mysteries, each chakra was said to be the seat of a *body*.[114] The first chakra or kundalini chakra, is the seat of the physical body, the generator of physical reality as each of us experiences it. In other words, the first chakra makes life. It makes all physical form: my physical form, your physical form, and others' physical forms as well. This chakra holds the very mystery of life (animated physical form) as well as the drive for procreation. Maintaining physical life is its most basic function.

Another term used for the first chakra is the root chakra. In Hindu, the first chakra is referred to as the muladhara chakra, a word derived from two words meaning "root" (mula) and "base" (adhara); it is thus the root, the foundation of the seven chakras.[115] We find our physical roots in the earth, so the first chakra, then, is the source of our groundedness as well as being our survival instinct.

The movement, the spinning of a chakra emanates a vibration. Because of the structure of our gonadal anatomy, however, the emanation of the first chakra cannot be monitored in the lab from the groin

114 Cf. note 28, Part One, Chapter Two. Annie Besant also discusses the subtle bodies of the chakra system (or "force-centres") in *Talks on the Path to Occultism*, op.cit., pp. 404-410. Yet another discussion of the chakras, specifically the kundalini or first chakra, can be found in *The Serpent Power* (*Shatchakra-Nirupana*) translated by Arthur Avalon, Madras, India: Ganesh & Co., available from Dover Publications Inc., 1974.

115 Motoyama, op. cit., p. 213.

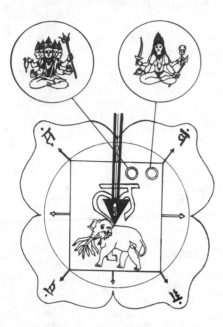

Fig. 2.1 THE MULADHARA CHAKRA. In Hindu tradition, this chakra is represented by a lotus with four crimson petals, each containing a golden Sanskrit letter. The associated female deity is the red-eyed Dakini. Her male counterpart is Ganesha, embodied in the form of an elephant. The inverted triangle symbolizes shakti, creative energy. Within the triangle sleeps the serpent, kundalini, coiled three and a half times around the Shiva linga. (Illustration from Swami Sivananda Radha's Kundalini: Yoga for the West, Porthill, Idaho: Timeless Books, 1981.)

[116] The Rolf Study.

area. In our research[116] we finally found a place on the back between the shoulder blades just under the heart where we could pick up the energy that came up the body from the first chakra. Otherwise, we would get radiation off the pubic bone and pick up hip joint and lower abdominal energies (see Appendix).

Anatomically, men and women have a first chakra placement which differs by almost two inches in the body. The first chakra is for the most part internal in a woman and is toward the surface of the body in a man. This is due to the influence of the respective male and female hormones, testosterone and estrogen. Testosterone pulls the chakra energies forward and down in a man, while the energies are pulled back and slightly up in a woman by estrogen. Ultimately what this means is there is a physiological difference in terms of how energy and information are processed through the pelvic region of each sex.

All the symbology of the first chakra is "in and out" symbology. It is movement symbology. It has serpentine motion. The energies or the vibrations that come into the body from the ground and make these undulating movements are the same vibrations that activate this center. If we breathe into those energies, if we move with them and if we are conscious of them, we will become aware that we have a first chakra.

It is important to always remember that movement and energy cannot be separated. The movement of energy in the body and physical movement (including its esoteric form) go hand in hand. Even when a healer is channeling and appears not to be moving, something is moving from the inside out as well as from the outside in. Thus, when we get into the area of the first chakra, the kundalini, we are always dealing with movement of some kind, usually the movement of vital energy or of life force itself.

Breath, Prana and Mind

Another name for this vital energy or life force is *prana* or *chi* (*ki*) energy. Breathing is the way of accessing prana. Prana and mind are also connected: prana probably accumulates and forms the mind, or the auric field (remembering that the aura and the mind are probably one and the same). Other things may make up mind too, but most certainly prana does.[117]

The connection between breath and prana is simple. Breath and prana enter the body simultaneously: breath, through the nose, and prana from the ground. If we inhale and let the body integrate whatever energy it can and then exhale and hold, the remaining prana will run back down into the ground.[118] Breathing is probably our conscious interface between matter (our body and air) and energy (prana and kundalini). It is the way we accumulate energy.

When we breathe, we should feel movement. Ideally we should feel breath from the hips, expansion in our trunk and breathing throughout the entire body, even in the feet. We should feel fully alive.

Kundalini and the Nervous System

Experiences are first recorded in the physical body, in the kundalini center, via the

[117] See Edward Rice, *Eastern Definitions*, New York: Doubleday & Company, Inc., 1980, p. 284. For the most ancient reference see the *Prasna*, the *Brihadaranyaka*, the *Taitttriya*, the *Chandogya* and the *Mahabharata Upanishads*.

[118] For a complete explanation of *Pranayama* or regulation of the breath (in Yoga practices), once more refer to the original source, the *Anugita*, Chapter VI, of the *Mahabharata Upanishad*. (Cited in Blavatasky, *The Secret Doctrine*, Vol. 1, p. 94.) For a summary, refer to Motoyama, op. cit. pp. 157-162.

nervous system. We know something has happened when we have a tactile sensation of it. In other words, to be physical, in the sense of the first chakra, is to have a nervous system or a way to tell the body what is occurring. In the first chakra, to be aware is to be tactile. Nothing happens until it happens in the first chakra; and nothing has happened until we sense it, until we feel it in a tactile way, until it touches us. Thus, for example, when any of us uses the metaphorical term, "That experience touched me deeply", we really mean that it registered in our first chakra. It registered all the way down to the physical body. Our interaction with our environment is dependent upon our own body's ability to simultaneously record and make us aware of the occurrence of some event or experience. Western medicine's definition of the body itself is only a part of the total reality. A complete view of the physical body must also include everything we sense about ourselves.

Therefore, we cannot discuss the kundalini without also discussing the nervous system. The kundalini is our primary means of sensing life and physical reality. Our secondary means is the nervous system, which transmits the energy of the experience or event first recorded by and in the kundalini to the brain via the spinal cord.[119] In this way the nervous system informs the body of the state of its vitality and health. If the kundalini is awake, our being will record the data, the experience. If the kundalini is not activated—if the serpent remains sleeping—the nervous system will still send a message to the brain, but we will not be able to recall the data or the event because it will not have been recorded; there will be no memory of the experience.

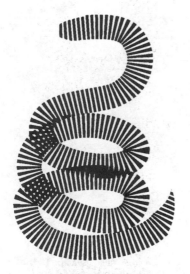

Fig. 2.2. *KUNDALINI, THE SLEEPING SNAKE.*

[119] The similarity between the image of the Ida and Pengali serpents winding their way up the central axis of the sushumna in the rising of the kundalini (see Fig. 2.3) and the spiral path of electrical currents up the spinal cord via the nervous system is not coincidental. The ancient sages were just as aware of the body's physiological nature as they were certain of the soul's temporary residence within it.

Not only is the kundalini the first place we have an awareness of the occurrence of an experience, but it is also the first place in which we can deny that anything has occurred. As long as we do not acknowledge that anything occurred, we do not have to deal with it. And we can avoid knowing that something is happening simply by holding our breath.

The kundalini is also the primary energy source for our spiritual vehicle. This means that people who do not have the "spiritual nervous system" (the chakra system) awakened are half alive. They are alive on the output; they are not alive on the intake. They feel only when they are active, only when they are "putting out"; they do not feel anything else. They live life in a numbed state. In some cases they live in a dangerously numbed state. This is how a person can have a cancer growing in his body and not know it or can have a kidney disease and not know it until the disease becomes so advanced that there are symptoms. To wait for symptoms is to wait for the secondary system, the nervous system, rather than the primary chakra system, to give feedback. By then it may be too late.

The Kundalini Awakening

While kundalini energy is not controlled by the genitals, it is related to hormones which are secreted by the endocrine glands of the reproductive organs. These particular hormones resonate in the frequency of red, and in not just one frequency but multiple frequencies, or harmonics. Remember from Part One that harmonics refers to multiple frequency bands

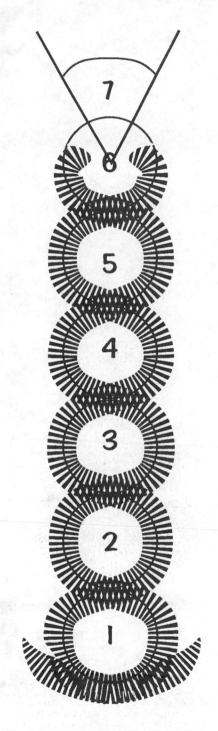

Fig. 2.3. THE KUNDALINI AWAKENED.

153

of the same color in a chakra. What this means then, is that everyone, including all the people that we think "don't have a root chakra", have one. It is true theirs might be in a lower or slower harmonic than the one we would like to feel in another person, but it is there nonetheless. This aspect accounts for the multiple kundalini openings that people on the path have throughout a lifetime. Each time we have an initiation or initiatory breakthrough or a peak experience, the kundalini opens in a new way—to the next frequency or harmonic of red.

The experience of "the rising" or the awakening of the "sleeping snake" of the kundalini can make us feel so incredibly alive because more energy is tangibly available to us than we have previously had access to. Right after the kundalini opens, the second chakra opens and connects to the third eye, so that everything we feel, we see. This is a highly visual state. The right and left hemispheres of the brain come into synchronization, and at this point, we are highly programmable.[120] Most importantly, when the kundalini opens, we have an activated awareness throughout the body. It is really alright to feel this alive, this aware, this good on a regular basis. That sensation is our life force moving through us, and it is very important, and it is very powerful. In his book *Theories of the Chakras*, Hiroshi Motoyama gives a personal and specific description of the awakening of his own kundalini.

> I was twenty-five years old. My early practice consisted of getting up at three a.m. every morning, practicing asanas for about half an hour, and sitting for three or four

[120] This process will be more fully discussed in Volumes Two and Six.

hours. The first part of the meditation was devoted to pranayama, the latter to the concentration on a specific chakra.

Here is the initial method of pranayama I practiced.

Inhale breath (prana) through the left nostril to the lower abdomen for about four seconds. Hold the prana in the inflated lower abdomen for eight seconds. Then raise the kundalini from the coccyx to the lower abdomen (the svadhishthana chakra) and contract the abdominal muscles. Visualize mixing and unifying the prana and the kundalini for eight seconds. Exhale through the right nostril for four seconds. One breath cycle, therefore, takes twenty-four seconds. Repeat the entire process, inhaling through the right nostril and exhaling through the left, and so on, alternately.

I performed this from fourteen to twenty-one times. After one or two months, I was able to prolong the period of kumbhaka (breath retention) to one or one and a half minutes. When I then concentrated on the svadhishthana or ajna chakra, worldly thoughts gradually ceased to enter my mind. I began to feel my body and mind fill with an extraordinary amount of energy.

As a result of the practice, my physical and psychological states began to show changes. I had often suffered from a stomach disorder and from an ear discharge. Also, I had been quite nervous and adversely affected both physically and mentally by bad weather. Within six months after I began yoga, these problems disappeared.

During continued practice, I began to notice some new sensations. I had an itchy feeling at the coccyx, a tingling feeling on the forehead and at the top of the head, and a feverish sensation in the lower abdomen. I could hear a sound something like the buzzing of bees around the coccyx. In ordinary daily life my sense of smell became so sensitive that I could not endure offensive odors.

These conditions continued for two or three months. One day, when I was meditating before the altar as usual, I felt particularly feverish in the lower abdomen and saw there a round blackish-red light like a ball of fire about to explode in the midst of a white vapor. Suddenly, an incredible power rushed through my spine to the top of the head and, though it lasted only a second or two, my body levitated off the floor a few centimeters. I was terrified. My whole body was burning, and a severe headache prevented me from doing anything all day. The feverish state continued for two or three days. I felt as if my head would explode with energy. Hitting myself around the "Brahman Gate" at the top of the head was the only thing that brought relief.

This, then, was the first time I had experienced the rising of the kundalini shakti to the top of my head through the sushumna. I did not experience as much physical or mental difficulty as is so often associated with this experience, probably because of the fortunate fact that my Brahman Gate was already open and the shakti was able to flow out into the astral dimension.[121]

We must keep in mind that this is only one example of kundalini awakening. Some people who open the kundalini inappropriately and at the wrong time or under bad advice often have a significantly painful experience because they are experiencing all of their resistance simultaneously with an energy flow that is trying to open. The resistance is what is so painful. Others who allow the kundalini to open spontaneously, but yet slowly, will usually feel little more than ripples of heat and rushes of energy. (Some of us have had initiations with various Eastern gurus, and we experienced heat flashes, as did Motoyama, for days afterwards.) This slower kundalini opening is probably more, certainly just as advantageous.

Hopefully, when the kundalini starts to open, we would have the faith to let it happen, as opposed to fighting it. People who report negative kundalini experiences—pain, heat, unconsciousness, loss of control, and so on—are not allowing themselves to fully feel. They are probably uncomfortable in their bodies and may even be tentative about being

[121] Motoyama, op. cit., pp. 240-41.

alive. For these reasons they attempt to "control" their experience.

It is important to remember that control and surrender are two points on a continuum and that if we try to control more and more, what ultimately happens is we finally break our resistance. We surrender. The more we control in one way—repressing sexuality, for example—the more the kundalini will be forced to open in another way, such as through anger. (All the chakras, in fact, are designed to function this way.) If, as part of a relaxation exercise, we physically tighten everything in the lower body, at some point we cannot hold that tautness any more, and suddenly everything becomes relaxed. The same is true of the flow of energy. If we try to hold onto it, at some point it bursts the dam and flows through. Thus, resistance does not in fact diminish our energy level; rather it serves to augment it. This is how the first chakra accesses energy in spite of resistance.

Many people become frightened by and will not allow themselves to experience the physical sensations of the kundalini awakening. Rather than trusting themselves and simply letting the body record the experience, they go directly to fear and stop the physical experience. Mistrust results in pain, which escalates the fear and triggers an attempt to control the experience. We might remember that if we give ourselves *permission* to control, we no longer need to *exercise* control. That is the really important issue when we start the process of trying to get extra power and extra energy to flow.

Breathing and Exercises for the Kundalini

If we are trying to open the kundalini, we must acquire a rhythm and flexibility in the hips. Generally, a forward and backward rocking motion is what is needed. Rocking chairs are useful for kundalini meditation because they help the pelvis to bend, to hold and to release, which is the kind of movement we desire. This kind of movement is vital to the breathing process.

I know of several exercises for opening the kundalini, each of which involves breathing, moving, concentration and awareness. Low tones, low frequencies and rhythmic sounds open the first chakra, which is why, in the native world, they use a heartbeat drum. All of this might seem esoteric until it is read on an oscilloscope. When we read the color red as it comes off the body on an oscilloscope, it looks like the heartbeat (see Fig. 2.4). Red is the only color that makes that long a wave pattern with such a high amplitude.

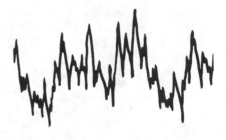

Fig. 2.4. RED WAVE FORMS. From The Rolf Study, oscilloscope printouts. Courtesy of Dr. Valerie Hunt.

Here is an exercise designed to assist you in feeling the *power* of kundalini energy. To do the exercise on the floor, try to sit comfortably but straight. If you prefer your favorite chair, please slide forward so that your back is erect.

When people begin to meditate, they often think they are hypnotizing themselves and worry about whether or not they conjured up their experience. If you start feeling *energies* while you are moving, you are likely to think that the *movement* is what you are feeling; therefore, do not move until you feel the *power* of the moving energies and let that power move you.

Begin by loosening your feet and knees. Wiggle around on your bottom until you know your body is alive. Then begin breathing gently until you feel a force of energy (or light or water) rise up through your feet. Let it move through your thighs, up into the core of the body.

Notice that if you bring a lot of energy up, the spine will start to gyrate. Your eyes do not have to be fully open, but try to keep them slightly open.

Gently turn your hands so they are palm up. Observe if any extra energy flows up through you and into your hands.

Next focus on what is happening in your head. If you start to feel at all lightheaded, reach up with your left hand and put it on top of your head. Then, let go. Notice that you could hold the energy in, and it would accumulate. You may feel heat in your face.

If you feel tension anywhere in your spine, bring in more energy, more power. Let it stay in the area that hurts or is tight, and allow the energy to rock there.

The following may seem very strange, but I suggest you try it anyway. Intentionally lean onto your right buttock, and try to do the above exercise. Then try it leaning on the left buttock. It is important if you think you are losing the sense of flow in the body, to throw yourself off center so you can feel the flow stop. Then recenter so you can distinguish between energy that is moving and energy that is not. At the point at which your body gets used to feeling this tactile sensation, test yourself. Lean forward, and see if you can block the sensation. Go back to your center. See what you feel. (The energy should be both more forceful and gentler.) Finally, sit back and be comfortable.

In most discussions of kundalini power we encounter the mistaken idea that this power is exclusive to a few people who have worked on themselves. Every athlete has to use this power. Every actor. Every musician. Every artist has to use kundalini power to keep himself fully conscious. The same is true for each one of us.

Kundalini and the Mysteries

In the ancient world the above exercise was used by all cultures on the planet as well as by the Egyptian, Greek, and Eleusinian Mystery Schools. These Mystery Schools used this exercise to make a person continually aware of his kundalini power. A Greek for instance who wanted to become a healer, could go to Epidauros and prepare to take the initiation there. The initiate would be placed in a subterranean snake-filled labyrinth for nine days without food or water. This exercise was the only thing that protected him from snakes. He had his own snake: his spine. The idea was to get a person to be a "snake" for nine days so that he would never lose his kundalini power thereafter.

All of the images of the Greek healer, Asklepios (Aesculapius), show him with snakes in his hands (see Fig. 2.5). Before Asklepios there were the Goddess mysteries which were discussed previously. The Goddess always wears the serpents around her wrists, her waist, her neck and her head, and sometimes many in her hair, an image which in mythology is represented in Medusa (see Fig. 2.6).

Medusa's power is that of the serpent scorned. It is an example of what can happen if we turn against the power that is Goddess

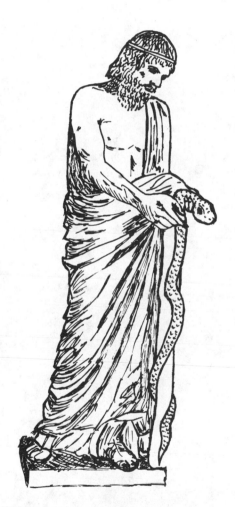

Fig. 2.5. *ASKLEPIOS, GOD OF HEALING. A.D. 2nd century Roman copy of a 5th century B.C. statue. Original in the Uffizi Museum, Florence, Italy.*

161

Fig. 2.6. THE HEAD OF MEDUSA. From a painting by Caravaggio. Courtesy of the Uffizi Gallery, Florence, Italy.

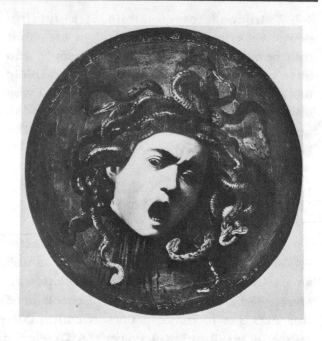

given: the look that kills. The power of the kundalini is projected through the eyes. I never cared what my mother, my grandmother or my great-grandmother said to me; I cared how they looked at me. We can look at someone to empower him, or we can do what my great-grandmother used to call "holding darkness", and thereby take power. She said that she would "hold darkness" because she did not think what I was doing was such a "bright idea". It was her way of taking power away from me before I did something wrong with it. We all still use that Goddess power whether we are conscious of it or not.

Kundalini Energy: Working on Two Channels Simultaneously

Consider energy coursing through the body or the process of channeling energy. People say, when they begin to sense energy, that they feel a "flow" or a "vibration" when

162

they put their hands on another's body. This awareness lasts for a minute or two. Then the system "ceases" to record any further data, and they are sure they have stopped transmitting or channeling energy. They did not stop channeling; they just stopped *feeling* it. This is primarily because our entire culture teaches us to think on only one channel. When we become more aware of the kundalini, our minds begin to work on two channels: we can *feel* whatever is coursing through us while we *think* about something else. The main purpose of the consciousness movement is (or at least should be) to make one "conscious": to enable one to think and feel on eight, nine, fifteen channels if possible, with awareness in all areas. This is precisely what the first chakra, the kundalini, is about: to awaken and stimulate conscious awareness on several levels at once and to open the flow of energy to several channels simultaneously.

Kundalini, Nervous Breakdowns and Meditation

All the myths about the rising of the kundalini and the accompanying loss of sanity are associated with the inability of an individual to hold awareness on several levels of reality simultaneously. Many of the states which we consider psychotic may in fact be "ecstatic". In both experiences, perception of reality alters. People have reported such phenomena as seeing lights or colors and hearing buzzing and ringing in the head. Some experience extremes of temperature as well as shaking of the body. There may even be a sensation of being lifted, as in levitation.

In addition, people who report kundalini experiences or the altered awareness of a kundalini "rise", almost always report experiencing two parts of themselves: the observer and the participant. These symptoms are identical to those of a nervous breakdown in which the nervous system short-circuits and the mind quits functioning altogether. There is a part of a person that is very rational which watches other parts of himself fragment, and there is no way to control the experience.

This "split" experience is often the culmination of a long series of events in a person's life in which one has been forced to focus on only one particular thing or level of reality. When a person is forced to think about only one thing at a time, the mind simply ceases to function effectively. Then, when a new channel of perceptual input is opened, as in a kundalini "rise", the "overstimulation" to the system can cause an "overload" of an already diminished capacity. This need not be a negative or fearful experience if one has learned in small steps how to operate in this larger way. People who meditate, for instance, learn to think on multiple channels and gradually begin processing all information with this broader understanding. Those who meditate regularly never go back to thinking the same way again.

First Chakra Energy in the American Culture

Suppression of the Life Force

Generally speaking, as Americans, the opening and the development of our first chakra has been inhibited by the "traditional" values of the dominant culture. For example, babies are very able to breathe with their whole bodies, to let their bellies flop and their buttocks relax, but by the time children reach approximately eighteen months of age, many of them have been conditioned not to breathe that way anymore. Our culture's puritanical influences are so pervasive as to have already begun to suppress these natural movements.

Also consider the fact that none of us was raised by parents who had seven open chakras. Our parents' chakras had their own particular harmonics and limited patterns. Thoughts (energy patterns) flowed from them through us, imprinting us with our parents' auric inventory. This is how, as children, we learn what behaviors are or are not "acceptable": what sensations, what feelings, what expressions. Often what is "unacceptable" develops into our own personal difficulties with the first chakra, such as the suppression of power, problems with sex and intimacy, repression of anger and lack of vitality.

Puberty is a particularly critical time in the development of the first chakra. Unfortunately, because of cultural mores and parental values, it can become a time in which the vital energies of the first center are further suppressed.

The hormonal changes of adolescence are ignited by the pituitary gland, which activates the entire endocrine system. As adolescents begin to develop secondary sexual characteristics, their behavior changes. They seem suddenly to acquire "independence". As they begin to realize and explore their physical and emotional needs, their attempts at self-expression are often looked upon with disapproval by parents and other authority figures. Such attempts at self-expression may even be completely prohibited by parents or other adults in authority. This is particularly evident with regard to the awakening sexuality of the adolescent. Touch, which is at best a "touchy" subject in our culture, often illicits a negative response from parents and teachers.

Adolescents also receive a great deal of nagging about "good posture": "Chest out, stomach in, buttocks tight". When the hips and pelvis are locked, energy flow becomes blocked. There is no sensation in that position. A person may be taller but certainly cannot feel. We begin suppressing this awareness, this sense of vitality, the need to touch, at the very time when it is the most powerful. This creates a backlog of suppressed energy which stays with many people throughout their entire lives and never finds an outlet.

Our culture specifically does not like women to manifest an open first chakra. We are told to stand, sit, move and walk in such a way as to restrict the natural rocking movements of the pelvis. The American ideal of beauty is a flat stomach and "tucked" buttocks. This results in a great deal of tension in the first chakra, so much so that most of us never have a sense of what it feels like to be relaxed in that area. I believe forceps are sometimes used in the birthing process because some women simply cannot "let go". They have held themselves so tightly and have repressed so much sexuality that they cannot achieve the openness and flexibility necessary at this most critical time.

From birth to adolescence and often through adulthood our culture discourages the open expression of first chakra energies. Often this suppressed power backs up so forcefully that a person begins to exhibit compulsive or obsessive behavior at an early age. Compulsive behavior is usually characterized by obsessional thinking or action. To a greater or lesser degree, a compulsive person frequently has a persistent or disturbing preoccupation with an often unreasonable idea or feeling.[122] Someone who feels a need to wash his hands dozens of times during the day could be said to manifest such compulsive behavior. One reason for such obsessive or compulsive behavior is precisely this stored-up, repressed power for which a person must find some outlet.

Addictions and the First Chakra

The other side of the compulsive personality is the addictive. It is not surprising that the American culture seems to have more than its fair share of both "compulsives" and addicts. The first chakra is connected to addictions, or, more precisely, to addictive behavior, in that addictions make us feel alive while at the same time they deaden us. They make us feel something other than what we are really feeling, something other than what we would feel without the distraction of the addiction. For example, if a person's addiction is to smoking then he would use tobacco to build a smoke screen (pardon the pun) between him and someone else. It makes him feel contained and numbs him to certain stimuli in his environment. It also suppresses the first center. While addictions can be found in all the chakras, they begin in the first. What the addictive personality needs to learn is how to feel something pleasant.

There is a lesson for every chakra. The lesson for the first chakra is "I feel; therefore I am". However, this does not refer to emotional feeling. It means "I sensate;

122 *The Merck Manual of Diagnosis and Therapy*, Thirteenth Edition, ed. by Robert Berkow, M.S., Rahway, New Jersey: Merck Sharp & Dohme Research Laboratories, 1977 pp. 1492-94.

therefore I am". As a result, if we do not give our bodies something to feel, particularly something that is "sensational", then this center is not going to be active. The problem becomes more acute the longer the energies of this chakra are suppressed. The longer the flow is blocked, the more likely the result will be some form of pathology.

Release of
Suppressed Energies and Fixations

We need to begin to work directly on the first chakra in order to release these suppressed energies. If the aura is anything, it is the mind: not the mind in the sense of the intellect but in the sense of the greater mind, the electromagnetic field which surrounds and generates the body.[123] Various frequencies of thought run in particular patterns around and through the body. Consequently, if one thought pattern persists habitually, the energy flow and, ultimately, the body itself begin to fixate and lock into a singular pattern of movement and behavior. This pattern in turn restricts the flow of thought and energy from exploring potentially alternate "positions". Other possible viewpoints cease to be supported by light and energy, and the whole system gets "stuck" in one pattern, one opinion, one reality. Any time one of our chakra centers is limited in its capacity to run in its own native patterns, for whatever reason, these fixations develop. Unfortunately, when we are fixated in our first chakra, the kundalini energy is limited, and our entire chakra system is detrimentally affected.

[123] See p. 207, Chapter Five. This mind-field phenomenon is further discussed in Volume Three.

Limitations of Too Little Kundalini

The kundalini is the primary energy source for our spiritual vehicle. If kundalini energy is limited, that limitation will be reflected in every part of our consciousness, until ultimately the realization of our spiritual path and our soul's journey down that path will be inhibited. If our first chakra is undeveloped, first and foremost our sense of touch, our sense of feeling is limited. The first chakra allows us to feel *ourselves* and to feel what we feel. This function is different from that of the second chakra, which is the seat of the emotional body and which allows us to sense what *others* are feeling. As a whole, our culture suffers from a condition of kundalini dysfunction: when the kundalini does not work in us, we do not feel who we are. Various levels of sensation and awareness are made possible simply by the *baseline*; the baseline is literally at the base of the spine and can be referred to as the base quantity of energy out of which any of us operates. If it is diminished in our system it will limit, first and foremost, our sex life: no libido.

The next capacity that is limited is our ability to perceive others. The kundalini center's function is providing energy or sourcing. If it is not developed and therefore lacks power, all our interactions are limited. For instance, the ability to perceive the quality and dimension of another's feelings is dependent upon how much of ourselves we feel with; if our own feeling level is very low, we will always perceive another's energy to be at maximum level, when, in reality, it is not.

Third, a diminished kundalini limits our intellect. We can only hold as much information as we can hold energy. Without kundalini we have neither a long term nor a

169

short term memory. A limited short term memory means *nothing* is stored. Consequently, when the kundalini flow is very diminished, trying to retrieve information from short term memory is very difficult. The mind is a field; therefore, it is everywhere. It is a vast and complex data base composed of many smaller energies (bits) stored throughout the tissues of the body.[124] It is the kundalini that allows a flow of energy to locate the information and bring that information up to the conscious level.

Diminished kundalini also affects the heart. It inhibits circulation and breathing. A limited kundalini restricts the warmth we feel toward others and the warmth and affection others feel toward us. In addition, it limits the awareness and expression of freedom in our lives. Without power, which originates in the kundalini, we have no sense of freedom, no awareness that it can be taken away and no ability to experience or express it in our day to day existence.

Next, a diminished kundalini inhibits the throat. No zip, no zing, no voice. No projection. The voice could be considered the kundalini for the spiritual center. The lower three centers, the physical, emotional and mental bodies, are replicated in a way in the upper three centers with the voice being the physical aspect of the spiritual world. In all creation myths sound or the voice or the word calls the earth into being.[125]

It is the kundalini which carries us from the three dimensional world into the next dimension. Once we enter the spiritual world, the kundalini manifests first as sound (fifth chakra) and then as light (sixth chakra). If there is little kundalini, there is little imagery, little visualization, lack of creativity and inspiration and no sense of the future.

124 See Part One, Chapter One.

125 Refer to Volume Five.

Finally and most importantly the last thing inhibited by diminished kundalini is the ability to move beyond physical reality through sleep, trance or other altered states. The crown chakra can be considered the gateway to the other world. When kundalini is diminished, the crown chakra does not have the power to open sufficiently to allow us "out" far enough to sleep peacefully. For those of us with sleep disturbances, the problem is often lack of power. Similarly, this lack of power can prevent us from reaching those states of consciousness wherein we reconnect to our Spiritual Source.

Chapter Three

FIRE POWER

Power and the Kundalini

Historically, each chakra is associated with a physical element. Fire is the element associated with the first chakra.[126] E v e r y color of the rainbow is contained in fire. Within the first chakra, all colors are visibly present, encompassed in red. There is a fiery quality, an incredibly beautiful translucent quality, that is the life force itself.

The first chakra is identified as well with the sun, the creator and sustainer of energy and life. This solar quality represents the male aspect of the first chakra in the same way that its lunar quality, symbolized by the snake, represents the kundalini and its feminine aspect. It is the solar flame which ignites passions, which begins and continues to create life. It is that which quickens and acts as the pilot light for the energy of the chakra system.

It is the red quality—the essence of fire —which sets all of the power in one's life. The red quality, the quality of our blood, the quality of our sexuality, the quality of our drive, the quality of our financial substance or prosperity all reside in the first chakra. When one is born, the body is grooved with a certain vital force (chi), and that vital force, that fire, is all the power in one's first chakra.

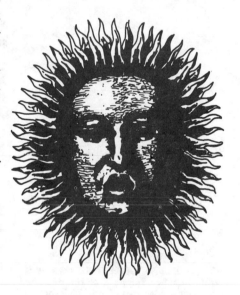

Fig. 3.1. SOLAR IMAGE.
From Montfoucon's Antiquities.

126 See Part Two, Chapter One.

173

Apparently, either through the birth process, through prenatal programming, or through life experience, a person may pull that power back and withhold it. This is particularly so if one has chosen to be born into a culture that does not take to first chakra activity. We as Americans presently live in a culture that is not very accepting of overt power, so we pull most of the power back. Nevertheless, our basic drive and ability to prosper reside in the first chakra, and how well we survive and prosper depends upon how much power we allow ourselves to have.

We need power in our spiritual lives as well. The fiery aspect of the first chakra is present in the indigo band appearing just before the white of the crown chakra. Mystical lore calls this fire the Flame of St. Germaine; it is that flame which the exorcist uses to remove (or neutralize) negativity. Without first chakra power, then, there can be no exorcism, no burning away of the negative.

Dual Qualities of the First Chakra: Powers of Spirit and Matter, Life and Death

• The first chakra, as do all the chakras, contains dual qualities which represent opposite potentials.[127] The dual qualities of the first chakra are spirit and matter, both of which relate directly to the fire element of this first center. In alchemical terms, matter becomes spirit and spirit becomes matter within the fiery crucible.[128]

The first chakra is the spiritual fire that manifests matter. At the moment of birth, spirit is fused into body as a baby passes through its mother's first chakra. It is

127 The "binary" aspect of the chakras is merely another example of the dualism which exists as a tenet of most philosophies and religious doctrines as well as those manifestations of nature, specifically the powers of attraction and repulsion present in electricity, magnetism and other force fields of which the chakra system is one.

128 For a summary of alchemy—its history, process and symbolism—refer to Hall, *The Secret Teachings of All Ages*, op. cit., pp. CLII-CLX. Of interest may be the origin of the root word "chem". As stated by Hall: "Khem was an ancient name for the land of Egypt; both ALCHEMY and CHEMISTRY are a perpetual reminder of the priority of Egypt's scientific knowledge." (p. CLII) Also see Pike, op. cit., pp. 772-800 for another summary of the evolution and symbolism of alchemy "a religion, a philosophy and a science which drew profoundly from the Kabbala".

the fire of the kundalini energies (both mother's and baby's) through which the spirit infuses life.

The first chakra transforms or burns data into pure emotion, the next frequency level. (The alchemical correspondence is the transformation of base metal into gold.) The first chakra can be trained to take all the kundalini power and transform it, discipline it, if you will, into pure emotion. Emotions must then also be trained and disciplined to have their true power. If this transformation does not occur, then every time anger is expressed, for example, there will be depression (an energy loss) instead of compassion (an energy gain).

When used in a conscious way, anger can actually trigger compassion. Once a person feels anger, he then knows what the next appropriate feeling or action should be. Consequently, any feeling can be taken right to the next stage, instead of being repressed, until finally compassion is attained. Anger is often the "match" which ignites the fiery flow of energy and sends it on its appropriate path up through the chakra system, creating higher and higher frequencies. But the anger must be in its pure form for this to happen. The biblical term for this kind of "pure" anger is "righteous".

The second dual components of the first chakra are the potentials of life and death. Where there is kundalini, there is life. Without kundalini there is the absence of physical life, which we call death. There is a continuation, a continuum, if you will, of consciousness, which runs through both these states. We are either *in* a body or *without* a body, but we always *are*. In the life cycle we are conscious of our moment-to-moment existence. In the death cycle, we are aware of what we have done throughout life, of how we have used our power.

Kundalini Power in the Ancient and Modern World: Charisma and Humility

In order to better understand first chakra power, we need to briefly explore what power means in the modern world and what it meant in the ancient world. Power in the ancient world was associated with personal magnetism. If we have very much of this kind of first chakra power, we will in fact be charismatic. This has nothing to do with attractiveness. It is associated with speaking with authority, dominating a room with energy; it is carriage. The charisma that certain movie and rock stars radiate is often called "animal magnetism", which is what first chakra power is in many ways. Whether "personal" or "animal", it is definitely magnetism.

With the exception of the entertainment industry and some areas of business enterprise, most contemporary Americans have difficulty acknowledging and using power appropriately. We actually suppress power by "sitting on it": it is very difficult to project personal magnetism from a seated position. Because of our Judaic-Christian roots, most specifically the Christian ideal of a humble carpenter who sacrificed his life for his fellow men, we often withhold power in favor of humility. This charisma-humility dichotomy exists in the first chakra.

Kundalini power is most definitely related to charisma. However, without humility, we become unbending. There is an important and relevant Buddhic teaching about power that reflects this charisma-humility dichotomy. That teaching states that one cannot be a pacifist until one has power, for unless one has power that he does not use badly, he is a coward, not a pacifist.[129] Without the power of the first chakra not only do we lack charisma; we also lack humility. If we refuse to take power, then whatever humility we display can only be false humility. However, when we take that power and begin using it, it strengthens and gives us flexibility. The knees bend fully, the legs extend fully, the hips rotate fully. Inversely, if we do not take that power and use it, the lower part of the body becomes stiff and inflexible.

That which we need the most and which has the most power for us is likely that of which we are most afraid. This fear reflects a denial of one's responsibility to be a fully active creator in the world, for it is the kundalini which makes us active creators. We should not be afraid of power; we cannot be afraid of using it. In fact, the power of the first chakra, if it is not used on some creative endeavor will diminish and may ultimately be extinguished. The fire component of the kundalini is our "starter" mechanism. Those who have had chronic disease such as rheumatoid arthritis or any of the dysfunctions that indicate the "starter" has gone out know how hard it is to recover from such illness. The body tries to "start" everywhere else; in the case of arthritis, it puts inflammation in the joints. That inflammation, however, does not produce the desired "fire power". The power has to be where it belongs—in the pilot light—or we cannot start the furnace. Without reclaiming power, there is little hope of conquering such diseases; if we are to reclaim our own power, then, we must "rise to the occasion" and allow the kundalini to come up the spine.

[129] One of the basic ideas underlying Buddhist philosophy is the duality of reality: one cannot know any one aspect unless he has also known its opposite. See Walpola Rahula, *Zen and the Taming of the Bull: Toward the Definition of Buddhist Thought*, New Jersey: Humanities Press International, 1978, which presents a clear discussion of the main tenets of Buddhism. Also refer to Nancy W. Ross, *Buddhism: A Way of Life and Thought*, New York: Knopf, Random House, 1980, which is a popular introduction to Buddhist thought and practice.

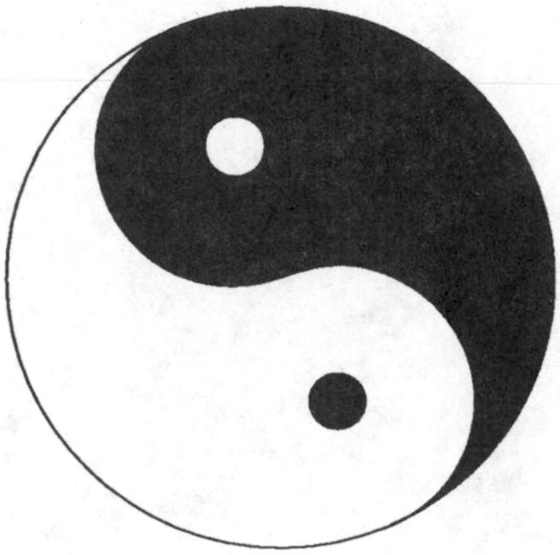

Yin and Yang Principle: Withholding and Reclaiming Power

All of Hindu and classical Zen literature is full of the principle of reclaiming power—taking whatever energy we are given and altering it to its opposite component.[130] For example, pleasure and rage are two coexisting potentials in the first chakra. By allowing ourselves to experience the ecstasy of "hedonistic" pleasure, we actually create the synaptical capacity for converting rage. Then when rage rises up within us, we can move that energy, that rage, into the pleasure center by tilting the pelvis slightly forward and moving the energy up. It is then used to regenerate our bodies instead of causing destruction. One of the classic Tibetan drawings of the chakras has a yin and yang in each chakra; this drawing is a precise representation of the refocusing of power and allowing it to turn back into its opposite, should one choose not to use it in its original form (see Fig. 3.2). In this way, there is no suppression of power. It is a much healthier process.

It often seems that there is no appropriate place for expressing many kinds of feelings. To avoid experiencing those feelings in the second chakra, many of us tend to hold back the power of the first. The result of this suppression is a first chakra that runs counter clockwise. By running this chakra backwards, we do not lose those unexpressed feelings but keep them suppressed. Thus, we do not have access to their power. In other words, instead of

Fig. 3.2. YIN-YANG.

130 Besides those texts already cited, see *Zen Flesh, Zen Bones*, ed. by Paul Reps, New York: Anchor, n.d.. This idea weaves its way through Reps' collection of Zen stories and Koans. Besides literature, most of the Oriental martial arts are based upon taking the opponent's energy and turning it against him. See Volume Two for further discussion of the yin and yang principle.

sending energy up the system, it is dissipated into the ground. We are losing a vast amount of energy and power. If we can turn the chakra around, then energy will again begin to flow appropriately, giving us access to our power once more.

Power is ours, but to understand it we have to use it. "Use it or lose it" is a contemporary adage which applies here. This cannot be an intellectual process; we have to *feel* the fire, use the power safely and wisely. We must be conscious of how and where we use it, and while doing so, we must also give that same life force back to others. We have to allow others their own power and their own use of it. Until each of us has more power, the success of one will threaten another. We can change this dynamic if, in our success, we empower others, particularly our friends, by giving them energy. This is the secret to energy work. We must always remember that the universe is the source of unlimited energy. This source is inexhaustible, and we can always tap into it to keep ourselves from being drained by others.

Using Power Appropriately

Power is not a four-letter word, but it might as well be. The mere mention of the word calls to mind negative images of greed, ambition, war, manipulation, corruption, dominance, subjugation, death and devastation. Both religious and secular literature is replete with teachings about the seductions and misuses of power. There is little historical allusion to the abundance and growth that can result from taking and holding power.

The underlying belief therein is that

the omniscient and omnipotent Deity is larger than we mortals and is *other than* or somehow *outside* us. The implication is that we are small, incomplete and undeserving; that somehow if we were to have power, we would likely misuse it and have to be punished for that misuse.

Certainly, our first attempts at using power might seem "sloppy". Mistakes are a natural part of the learning process. The fear of misusing power is very real at the personal level as well as at the political and global levels. For decades now many of us have criticized those in positions of power. We have challenged the "powers that be" and have repeatedly witnessed the demise of political and religious leaders of questionable integrity. We are, however, reluctant to place ourselves in such positions. We refuse to *take* power or leadership as though we fear duplicating the behavior of those we criticize. We fear being corrupted or else being perceived as threatening. It is my view that it is useless to criticize those in power unless we are willing to involve ourselves, to participate in the operation and the management of things. *Not using* power is in itself a misuse of power. It is not good for the body, nor does it help to change the world. Until we take the power that is our birthright, we will be threatened by others who have power. Until we learn to use power appropriately, we will potentially be perceived as a threat.

We must learn to walk in the world as a *Bodhisattva*.[131] A Bodhisattva uses power without others being aware that he is doing so. Ultimately, when we have practiced taking and using power, we will do it so well that others will not feel threatened by us. In time, with practice, we become "warriors", capable of fighting for an honorable peace or a

---

[131] A *Bodhisattva*, in Buddhism, is a person who has attained great moral and spiritual wisdom, especially one who rejects nirvana in order to assist mankind.

lasting healing. Once we understand that this power is with us, the security that it gives us keeps us from making harmful mistakes.

In the New Age the idea that each of us is an expression of Deity implies that the empowerment of the individual must include an acknowledgment of a relationship to all other sentient beings, each of whom is also a part of God. This idea and acknowledgment paves the way for the individual to express his divinity, to feel empowered and deserving, in other words, to take power and use power and thus manifest a better life experience.

Our intention becomes very clear when we understand that, whether we are conscious of it or not, we influence our environment. For example, when I began to understand that my aura—my energy field—controlled whether plants lived or died in my home, I began to further see that my aura also affected the way my pets lived, the way my children lived, the way my neighbors lived. To have power is to have impact on everything around us. We can learn not to fear that impact but to use it—consistently, consciously and responsibly—integrating it in a natural way into our daily living. If each of us were self-responsible for having more power, for carrying more light, more love and more wisdom, then surely the planet would be a better place.

The Need for Power in Service

One last aspect of power deserves consideration: power and its relation to service. We must reconcile the need for power and charisma with the desire and the necessity for service. The capacity to serve requires a reasonably secure level of power.

In order to take care of another person we must have at least enough power to allow an individual to feel safe in our presence. If we do not have that amount of energy, or if we have less energy than the people we seek to serve, we are going to be taking from them in spite of ourselves and our intention to give. We have to be able to pull spiritual promise through us "on command", or our giving will be less than we want it to be.

Not only must we be willing and able to share of ourselves in this way, but we must also have enough energy to "pull in" that which supports us on our path. In giving, we open the flows that feed us. We must learn to give from the source which is infinite in supply, and thus avoid depletion and burn out. We must learn to channel the energy of giving rather than drawing on our own life force, and to place that giving ahead of other considerations or limitations.

Finally, we cannot serve unless we have an awareness of our physicality. It is only through a healthy relationship with our first chakra that we may serve most fully and discover that service is indeed the path back to our cosmic beginning. It is the way back to Deity.

Kundalini and Prosperity

It is interesting to note that the American culture has elected to make money green. Green is, of course, the complementary color of red; the power behind prosperity is the red frequency of the first chakra. The ability to attract, which is the essence of prosperity, is directly related to the power of one's aura. The larger the aura, the greater the capacity to attract and hold.

Whether one attracts randomly or specifically, one brings something to oneself; should we not direct our attractive field, we are likely to attract people who need aura, who are simply needy and want us to care for them.

It would seem, therefore, to be a good idea to be more selective about what we seek to attract. But many people who see themselves as being on a spiritual path also see an apparent conflict between that path and material prosperity. They are unaware that it is the ethical status of the person seeking material prosperity which matters, not the money itself. They miss the point that money should be regarded simply as another form of energy which needs to be utilized and exchanged. Finally, they ignore a basic reality: in order truly to be generous with one another, we require whatever level of prosperity allows us such generosity.

It is a basic law of prosperity that if we spend money, we get it. If we spend what we have on what we need to serve others and to serve God, it is replaced instantly. The greater our capacity to give, the greater our likelihood of security. It is in attachment to acquiring prosperity, then, that we lose sight of the reason to attract in the first place, and it is there that the conflict between material gain and spirituality really arises. Energy, and prosperity, must be reciprocal.

Chapter Four

SEXUALITY, KUNDALINI AND KARMA

Sexuality: Exchange

People exchange energy in many ways. Anytime there is an energy exchange of some kind, there is sexuality. Energy, by virtue of its electromagnetic nature, has a positive and negative flow. This back and forth movement or rhythm, this ebb and flow, registers in our bodies as sexual. Thus, our culture tends to interpret many types of interaction as sexuality. The primal life force, the energy of creation, blood, "fire", power, survival—all vibrate within the red frequency band. Because this frequency band is the kundalini, the body has an awareness of these interactions on a physical level. Furthermore, there is a sense of anticipation, a feeling of excitement with every energy exchange, which further confuses the system, since these feelings are also associated with arousal. We must keep in mind that when energy is moving, and we feel it moving, it is not an indication that sexuality is the next step. It is an indication that every part of us is alive.

To the degree that the first chakra is open, one will be tactilely aware and feel alive. When the kundalini is flowing, one has a powerful physical presence and impact on others. Then it is often said that one has "charisma". Some people who carry this quantity and quality of energy are frequently misunderstood and considered to be overly sexual or too sensual by a society born of a Puritanical consciousness. Life force is life force. In energy terms, there is little difference between the life force of artistic creation and that of procreation, between the power needed to give life to a child and that needed to create a political system or even to give birth to a spiritual path.

Orgasm:
Empowerment and Mergence

In any energy exchange, the *quality* of energy is important. But it is the *quantity* of energy which determines the level of openness and expansion one is able to attain. Orgasm requires an open and expanded state. It does not occur in the first chakra; kundalini energy must travel up nearly the entire chakra system to the third eye in order to stimulate the neurotransmitters in the brain responsible for the experience of orgasm. This requires an abundance of energy, a quantity of energy beyond the usual amount necessary to sustain us through our daily activities and interactions.

The exchange of energy in lovemaking is an aspect of the first chakra, the true purpose of which has long been mis-understood. Orgasm is a trance-like state; the purpose of sexuality is the expansion and empowerment of one's partner through an exchange of energy. Often what is conscious in one partner lies hidden in the other. The partner's energy has the power to ignite in us those aspects of ourselves previously unexplored. The beauty and function of sexual intimacy is in encompassing the "opposite", in becoming more than we are alone. Sexuality allows every living being to know that there is "other" and that mergence with that other is possible; that all of us can attain, even briefly, One Mind.

The quality of this mergence is dependent upon how much energy we can accumulate and hold in our system. The Oriental sexual practice of *kamasutra*[132] is designed to access this greater energy. In the union of *kamasutra*, the partners open the feeder systems in the legs, arms, the jaws and above the ears, and if the *kamasutra* technique is mastered, the hundred or so secondary chakras in the body are also opened. This makes an enormous amount of energy available to the couple.

The quality of one's sex life, of how well we merge, also depends upon how well one can communicate with one's partner. Communication needs to be verbal, nonverbal and tactile. Ultimately quality again depends upon quantity: one must be able to move enough energy to put the partner into a trance, an altered and higher state of consciousness. If, for example, one stimulates the partner but does not put him or her into a trance, the result is not orgasm but an anxious state in which performance becomes impossible for either partner, male or female. Trance-like states are tidal; they ebb and flow, push and pull. Without a rhythm, communication, or abundant energy, there can be no altered state—no orgasm.

For orgasm to occur, one must first learn to master the undulating movement of the kundalini energy. One must know when

132 *The Kama-Sutra*, C. 300 A.D., (English translation, *The Kama Sutra of Vatsyayana* by Sir Richard Burton, 1883) has been described as a Hindu love manual. It is actually a distinguished treatise on love and pleasure intended as a technical guide to sexual enjoyments utilizing music, perfume and lyric poetry as auxiliary sensual aids. It is also a realistic presentation of amatory relations between the sexes in ancient India. (*Encyclopaedia Britannica*, Vol. 13, 1985, p. 26).

to move or push the energy and when to surrender, when to release and pull the partner's energy. Both the first and second chakras are involved in this process, both "fire" and "water". This probably accounts for the discrepancy among existing chakra texts as to whether sexuality resides in the first or the second chakra. What is so is that during sexual intimacy, energy must leave one's first chakra and enter the partner's second chakra. Furthermore, this must be a reciprocal process. Besides the obligation to give, there is an obligation to surrender. In sexual intimacy, if one does not surrender, there is no true exchange and therefore no orgasm.

In the final analysis, one's ability to achieve orgasm is not dependent upon one's partner. Rather, the experience is limited by an individual's issues around sexuality. If sex is associated with violation or coercion, achievement of mergence with another will be next to impossible. If the experience of oneness is associated with a particular kind of sexual encounter, response might be inhibited simply because the "ideal" circumstances will never be repeated. Ultimately, the degree to which one is able to achieve sacred mergence with another is related to the limitations—physical, emotional or mental—placed on that union. The quality and quantity of energy necessary for a complete and fulfilling sexual experience is essentially dependent upon one's views and experiences of sexuality.

Orgasm: A Trance State

The mergence or oneness of sexuality is intended to be a heightened awareness, not a deadening, a numbing or a sleep state.

Besides empowerment and mergence, the goal of sexuality is to enter and maintain a simultaneous state of deep relaxation and expanded consciousness. In our culture relaxation usually means sleep; people go to sleep rather than becoming more awake. A common experience after engaging in sex is to fall asleep. Contrary to some popular thought, when one is "exhausted", when one has little or no energy, sleep is not possible. For sleep to occur, there must be sufficient energy to allow the astral body to leave the physical body. In sexual intimacy, once the agitated energy is transformed through orgasm, the energy accessed is abundant enough to allow this to occur. This is fine for the physical body. However, we would grow more in power and consciousness if we "stayed in" the body, stayed present, as the energy expands and increases.

Orgasm is defined as an "organism or an orgasmic experience in which two units function as one".[133] It is the sense of being a single organism, a single cell. The ideal of sexual intimacy is to stay in that "single-celled" feeling, that heightened state of consciousness, for as long as possible. This expanded trance-like state lasts only as long as energy can be held and not released from the system. Sexual partners can assist each other in maintaining energy—and thus extend orgasm—by preventing the kundalini energy from leaving the other's system. This can be done by placing one's hands on the partner's back to direct the energy flow as well as by holding those areas where energy tends to "leak out". One can keep one's mate in the body—and thus maintain the energy in the region of the third eye—by putting his or her hand on top of the other's head.

[133] *Webster's Seventh New Collegiate Dictionary.*

The emptiness one frequently feels after making love is indicative of an inability to stay in the expanded state long enough to produce neurotransmitter activity in the brain, of a failure to maintain that "single-celled" feeling. Once again, the quantity of energy one is capable of carrying determines the depth and quality of the sexual experience. If one's usual energy field is rather small, the extra energy accumulated during sexual activity will likely be too much for the system to process, resulting in a "loss of consciousness" as one is pushed out of the body. The minute the energy accumulated during sex puts one to sleep, the meaning of the experience, the feeling of oneness, of empowerment, the potential for growth and consciousness, has been lost. Once this happens, there is a constant need to merge again, a feeling of loss and separation as partners pull apart from each other.

On the other hand, the desire to mate over and over again within a brief period of time does not necessarily imply that the sexual experience has been unsatisfactory. More than anything else, it is an indication that the open, expanded state achieved in the sexual mergence has been so pleasurable, so "awakening", that one desires and seeks to remain in that heightened state.

Similarly, the sadness which is sometimes experienced at the conclusion of lovemaking springs from the fear that one will not be able to experience that special union, that feeling of complete mergence again. Some misinterpret this feeling and seek to duplicate their last "fulfilling" sexual experience in the belief that the pleasure they felt is intrinsic to a particular set of circumstances. The reality is that "good" sex is not a single experience one attempts to replicate until boredom sets in; sexuality must involve time, place, proximity and multiple experiences. Most importantly, "good" sex means having an open system, a body capable of maintaining a high level of energy exchange and a willingness to explore the deeper mysteries of oneself through another.

Sexuality and the Spiritual: Mergence With Deity

In spiritual practice, a great fear has always been that one will use one's sexuality in an unspiritual way. This fear has been the source of most of the negative literature regarding the first chakra and kundalini power. The issue is further complicated when we examine major religious cultures and find celibacy as a spiritual discipline practiced within the various priesthoods. It is as if one cannot be sexual and spiritual at the same time. This is simply not so.

Celibacy in its most basic sense can be considered a "mating" with one's god. The intent of a vow of celibacy is presumably to free oneself to merge exclusively with deity. One enters into divine intercourse, as it were. Underlying the practice of celibacy is a belief that in order to maintain this exclusive union with God, it is necessary for one to remain "clean" and separate from those human desires which distract one from the ultimate goal of divine union. Since sexuality in its procreative sense is considered to be the beginning of all that is human, of all human desires, it is to be avoided. By remaining "clean", free from the "taint" of humanity, it is believed one can better sense and recognize the divine. Thus come the admonitions about the "evils" of sexuality and of the kundalini itself.

In the exercise of celibacy among the Eastern religious sects, the kundalini is not shut down. The flow which originates in the earth and rises upward is not denied. However, the choice is made not to exchange energy with another but instead to conserve it for the purpose of achieving an experience of the deity. This is not true of celibacy as it is practiced in the West, however. Western religion has made Satan's abode below, underground, so to speak. Therefore, so as not to allow Satan into one's life, that flow which comes from the earth has been blocked; the first chakra has been shut down. In cutting us off from the earth's electromagnetic flow, this belief has resulted in a lack of "groundedness" both in celibacy as it exists in Western religion, and in Christianity itself. In Eastern religious practice, it is believed that the earth is as sacred as the heavens; there is no Satanic force abiding below. Thus, there is neither the necessity nor the desire to close off the earth's energies or the kundalini.

All of the powers of the kundalini relate to mergence with another and thus to mergence with God. Each time we use sexuality to separate us from another, to avoid responsibilities or to numb ourselves in some way, then we have "sinned" against that power. We have "missed the mark",[134] we have missed the opportunity to reconnect with the Oneness, to experience, however briefly, the sense of union with God.

134 The Egyptian glyph for sin was a target. To them sin simply meant "missing the mark". A bull's eye indicated the conquest over sin, "hitting the mark".

Sexuality and Service

Sexuality is part of the rest and regeneration cycle of those who live on this planet. Sexuality becomes particularly essential to those in service because by and large they will be spending most of their lives in the presence of negative energy fields— disease, depression, addiction. If people who serve do not stay "filled up", those negative fields will attach to them. When kundalini is not flowing and the field is depleted, a vacuum is created. Such a field will tend to attract other fields of greater or larger energy. If we are constantly around negative fields, those fields will impact us. When people are tired, when their energy feeder systems are closed, when they are out of their bodies, they are fair game for all the negativity around them. The obvious way to avoid such situations is to be open enough to keep the kundalini always flowing, the system always conscious.

Sexual activity is an opportunity for each of us to access this energy and consciousness. The sexual ideal is an open system, capable of taking in, processing and exchanging an abundance of energy. In fact, one's sexual pattern—how one accesses and exchanges energy in sexuality—will be reflected in every other aspect of one's life. Put another way, kundalini energy is basic to every success in life: health, business, relationship and service. Without kundalini energy moving through the system, one is unable to impact any person or circumstance enough to manifest any change, desire or success.

When reference is made to being "open" and being "present", what is meant is

193

that kundalini energy is flowing and the level of energy exchange is high enough that one is aware of the kind of energy and experience entering his field—positive, negative or indifferent. That consciousness in turn enables us to push negativity out of the system, to eliminate that which is unhealthy or undesired and to retain that which is healthy and desirable. With such awareness there is safety: while a person may not be protected from *taking in* negativity, he is able to *recognize* it and may then *eliminate* it from his energy field.

Some people try to protect themselves from harmful or negative fields by surrounding themselves in white light. The problem with this technique is that white light functions to keep out all energy, both negative and positive. This inhibits change and thereby restricts one to whatever consciousness he possesses at the time. While this is less than ideal for anyone, for those in service to others, this is a particularly unacceptable position. We must be willing to change. For each of us the goal must be to become ever more exquisite, open and delicate in our perceptions. This quality of perception—this awareness—is dependent upon the power and the openness of the kundalini.

The Kundalini Center and Karma

Whether it is within the act of mergence in sexuality or by means of the rising kundalini of sacred initiation, the purpose of the first chakra and first chakra energies is awareness: awareness not only of our own life force as it moves through us, but an awareness of our connection to that Force which creates and maintains life throughout the entire universe. As the chakra which allows us this awareness, the first center is the main chakra in which our karmic journey begins.

Karma is usually defined as both action and the results that action brings.[135] Every activity brings with it certain consequences, and according to this idea, our lives are influenced (through our subconscious tendencies) by our past actions (including those of past incarnations).[136] Relative to this, each new action creates new *karma*. As *karma* is either "made" or "paid", there are lessons to be learned in the process. Without the awareness provided by the first chakra, those lessons would slip by unrecognized. In other words, as the energies move from the feet through the kundalini center and up the spine, it is this first center that determines whether or not we can stay conscious long enough to understand the point—the lesson—of whatever is occurring.

Until this kundalini center is more open, some of the changes we want cannot be manifested because we simply run out of energy. How much energy we have affects how well we can change, how well we can learn our karmic lessons, how quickly and effectively we can move through our karmic patterns and bring our soul ever closer to its evolutionary goal.[137]

[135] James Fadiman and Robert Frager, *Personality and Personal Growth*, New York: Harper & Row, Publishers, Inc., 1976, p. 398.

[136] Ibid.

[137] See Volume Two for a more thorough discussion of *karma*.

Chapter Five

SCIENCE
AND THE CHAKRAS

The Rolf Study

While it can never be proven that the first chakra is the center wherein one's karmic journey begins, the reality, the energies and the relation of this first center to one's vitality and survival are more than simple theory. In the mid-seventies, Dr. Valerie Hunt conducted a research project at UCLA which studied the effects of Structural Integration or rolfing[138] on neuromuscular structure, emotions and the energy field itself. The results of this study provided evidence not only that the red frequency of the first chakra exists but that it is connected in a very real way to an awareness of physical sensation. More than that, this research presented empirical data regarding the frequencies and actual functionings of all the chakras.[139]

Briefly: Subjects were asked to lie on a table where they were to participate in a rolfing process. The area of the research in which I took part involved the study of the effects of rolfing on the energy field. Electrodes were placed over major chakra and acupuncture locations on the subject's body, with EEG electrodes positioned on the head. Then, during the session, I read both

[138] Rolfing is the name commonly given to Structural Integration, a system of reshaping and realigning body posture through deep (and sometimes painful) stretching of the muscle fascia accomplished by direct, deep manipulation. Its founder was Ida Rolf, from whom it receives its more familiar name.

[139] Cf. Part One and Appendix.

197

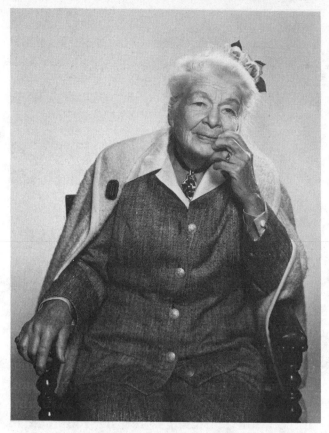

the subject's and rolfer's auras and recorded any changes in color, shape or movement of the fields as I observed them. Simultaneously, the frequencies of the electromagnetic radiation emitted from the subject's body during the course of the session were recorded on an oscilloscope, which was being monitored by Dr. Hunt in a separate enclosed instrument room. The process was specifically described by one of our participants, himself a scientist:

> The UCLA Rolf study, which began in January 1975, demonstrated that deep rolfing massage results in pronounced changes in the electrophysical activity of muscles. Of even greater significance were the

findings of changes in the body's energy field or aura. The energy field was described by Rev. Rosalyn Bruyere while Dr. Valerie Hunt simultaneously recorded electrophysical activity from the body. To the amazement of all concerned, the two correlated with each other. As a research scientist, I found it interesting to be a participant-observer in this whole process—serving as a subject being examined and listening in as a scientist to each day's discoveries.

At the Movement Behavior Laboratory at the Kinesiology Department, Dr. Hunt and her assistants applied electrodes to various areas of my body. The two rolfers in the study then alternated with each other for each of the ten sessions I was being monitored, and Rosalyn read the aura while Valerie stood in her physiological recording booth. Most of the rolfing sessions began with some manipulation of the hands or feet and ended with an adjustment of the neck, shoulders, spine and pelvis. At the time I did not know much about chakras, acupuncture meridians, or the flow of psychic energy, but I did experience a warm, tingly, spacy feeling soon after the rolfer laid his hands on me and began the deep massage. I experience similar sensations when I meditate or am hypnotized. Rosalyn found that when subjects reported spacy feelings, their auras showed more activity in the throat, third eye, and crown chakras and decreased activity in the legs. Dr. Hunt's recordings showed a parallel pattern. In the early sessions, I also had a lot of anxiety about how painful the rolfing would be, at which times the energy field activity was highest in the heart and throat chakras.

Auric analysis of pain and anxiety was probably one of the most fascinating results of the rolf study. At times, the rolfer's hands move over long stretches of muscle and there is a strong burning sensation. When a rolfer comes to an area where muscles are knotted or inappropriately bound together, he applies a very deep massage with his knuckles, fists or elbows. This can lead to extremely intense pain. At times I would think, "That wasn't as bad as I thought it would be," whereas at other times my anxiety raced through my mind and I would think, "What have I gotten myself in for?" Although it wasn't technically feasible to record physiologically from the actual muscle site being manipulated, Rosalyn did observe that a flash of red appeared over the areas of the body where the subject was experiencing pain from rolfing. When the deep massage was continued, the first chakra red wave forms shifted back and forth to orange which is the color of the emotionally related second chakra. Emotional processing went on for some time. Yellow, on the other hand, was observed when subjects dealt with their experience intellectually, trying to overcome pain with their will. The color green, related to transition and loving, was rarely seen in this study. Blue became evident when the subjects recalled early life experiences and violet wave-forms were higher in amplitude when the subjects were imaging an experience. The violet would shift from the third eye to the throat and back up to the third eye just before the subject reported they were picturing something. There was often a pluming of white light at the crown chakra at the same time. The aura was pure white when the subjects reported they were in a higher state of consciousness.

The rolfer's hands and arms usually carried a large blue or white corona but when subjects reported pain (Kundalini red), the rolfer's aura suddenly changed to a violet pink (the color of empathetic, spiritual loving), and this tended to calm the subject's field. After the first few sessions, the subjects seemed less affected by the pain of rolfing. Red was absent from their field and muscular flinching and wincing lessened. They flowed with the pain as they accepted the soothing violet of the rolfers.

Even though the colors of the seven chakras of the body have been variously described by psychics for centuries, the rolf study was the first time these colors were specifically related to certain frequencies of electrophysiological recordings. The primary colors were found to be red, yellow and blue. These are the colors of the first (Kundalini), third (adrenal or solar plexus), and fifth (throat) chakras. The respective physiological frequencies related to these three colors were waveforms with bandwidths of 640 to 800 Hertz (cycles per second), 400 to 600 Hertz, and 100 to 240 Hertz... In Fourier analysis[140] the pattern of the red waveform was that of irregular groupings of short spikes, whereas yellow resembled a smooth, round sine wave and blue exhibited large sharp peaks and troughs with small deflections riding upon them. In audio recordings red sounded like a siren, yellow like a musical tone, and blue like a rumble. The secondary colors, orange, green and violet related to the second (abdominal), fourth (heart), and sixth (third eye) chakras. Physiological frequency recordings showed that orange was a combination of the frequencies of red and yellow, green was made up of yellow and blue waveforms, and violet brought together the high frequencies of red with the low frequencies of blue. The white corona seen at the crown chakra was a combination of all frequencies just as in the color spectrum[141] (see figures included with Appendix).

[140] Fourier analysis, named for Joseph Fourier (1768-1830), its formulator, is a mathematical process of analyzing the conduction of heat in solid bodies. In our study, reproductions of pure color wave forms were made using a Viomation Transient Recorder No. 802 to store the wave form and expand and project it on an oscilloscope for photography. Raw data samples of the wave forms manifested in our rolfing process were further processed by Fourier analysis using a Techtronic 7L5 Spectrum Analyzer. Photographs were then made of these frequency spectra displayed on a Techtronic 7603 oscilloscope.

[141] Terry Oleson, Phd., "The Rolf Study: An Analysis of Auras" as printed in *The Light Bearer*, Vol. 10, no. 4., April, 1985.

Red on the Oscilloscope

When we explore the red frequency on an oscilloscope, it looks like continuing spirals connected by sine waves, a continuous flaring, an irregular grouping of short spikes (see Fig. 5.2). (Metaphorically speaking, the sine wave could be considered the "snake" within the red frequency band.) The red wave pattern on the oscilloscope actually demonstrates how red energy flows. When working with energy, most healers tend to run non-cyclical energy, i.e. direct current.[142] What direct red current does is produce a roller coaster effect; there is an increase, followed by a decrease of energy flow (which is what the sine wave represents). Then the pattern repeats itself. I believe it is the decrease in energy flow (which tends to feel like downward movement or a sensation of falling) that frightens everybody: we no more get a rush of red than we experience a "sinking" sensation. That is also the sensation we feel in an experience such as anger. Anger produces the same effect when it flashes. It rises up, and then moves through a depression and then rises again. This cycle is very natural: life's high times are usually followed by periods of relative stasis which are followed by crisis, which are followed by another period of stasis, and so on.

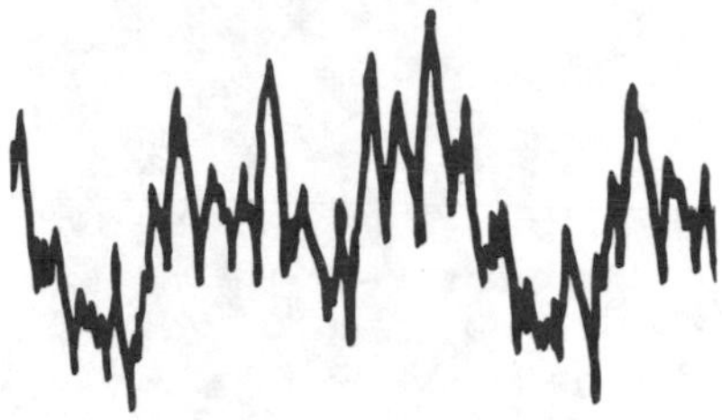

Fig. 5.2. RED. A red wave form as recorded by the oscilloscope. From The Rolf Study, *courtesy of Dr. Valerie Hunt.*

Red in Rolfing and Healing

During my years of research I saw a great amount of yellow in the first and second chakras. However, during the rolfing itself I saw only red in the first chakra. Thus it

[142] Cf. Part One, Chapter Four.

203

would seem that when someone gets into pain, the first chakra cries for "life". The late Ida Rolf herself said that pain was overrated. Pain is not the purpose of rolfing. The drawing forth of the life force itself is what is important in rolfing. Healing energy must have at least a carrier band of this life sustaining red frequency. For one thing, it is needed to make red blood cells. To dissolve calcium also takes red—powerful, hot red. Most healers I know heal in purple, which combines the powerful regenerative red frequency with the "cooler", soothing blue.

One of the results of running energy on a person is vasodilation, which is why people flush when they undergo a healing treatment. Another result is an increase in blood perfusion. Both these phenomena are related to the movement of red energy in a body. One of my mentors channeled red energy between the first and second center to stimulate the system. In other words, he used his kundalini energy to tap into another's. When the system is stimulated in this way, kundalini energy flows from the point of stimulation directly into the heart chamber. Since blood perfusion is increased, the heart muscles relax. This rising kundalini flow also causes one to go into an altered state of consciousness, and the heart chakra opens.

The DC Shift

We were fortunate enough to have recorded this process in our research. In one of our rolfing sessions I observed red energy flow to the heart of a woman subject. As soon as the energy arrived at the heart center, it looked to me as though the heart had "popped". When this happened, the woman's normal tired yellow aura seemed to immediately turn white and expand to about two feet around her body. This is what I saw in the aura and what the oscilloscope confirmed. Simultaneous with my seeing the "pop", all the electrodes reported white. On an oscilloscope white looks like all frequencies at once (see Fig. 5.3). The scope simply filled up with all frequencies simultaneously. I recall the subject reporting:

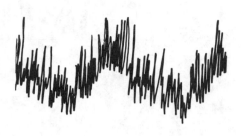

Fig. 5.3. WHITE. White as seen by the oscilloscope. From The Rolf Study, *courtesy of Dr. Valerie Hunt.*

> I don't know what's going on. I'm floating over my body. I can see everything below me, but I'm not looking that way. I can't move my hands, I'm not in touch with my body, but I can feel my body. I can feel all of my body; I've never felt all of my body before. How can I feel my body if I'm not in my body?

While what we recorded was the "opening" of a heart chakra, when the data was more closely examined, we realized that the implications of the event and the process were even more significant. The process we recorded was actually the rising of the kundalini. What I thought I had observed was the subject's aura expanding from a normal, rather tired appearance to a huge white aura almost instantaneously. However, the process did not really happen that directly. When we did a detailed analysis of the data, we discovered that the shift had happened so quickly that I had missed a very important stage. The yellow aura had not immediately transformed to white. It had first spread out into blue before tripling in amplitude and then turning white. What had been captured on the equipment was the process of an altering

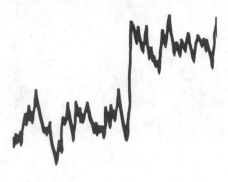

Fig. 5.4. DC SHIFT. A DC Shift as seen by the oscilloscope.

consciousness. This phenomenon suggests what happens when the kundalini moves fast enough to overtake all the other electrical processes of the body: one is in fact projected into an altered state of consciousness.

Our subsequent studies further revealed interesting information about the kundalini. The more exhausted and more stressed we become, the more likely we are to experience the altered state, or, to use the vernacular, to have a "peak" experience.[143] This is contrary to what we are often taught by meditation teachers, who tell us that in order to "open" ourselves, we need to relax more completely so as to gain more energy. We also learned that if, when the kundalini rises, we "change gears" or shift mental focus, our energy shifts back down, and we lose the altered state.

During an altered state, the aura is expanded and thick, which is different from an intoxicated or drugged state in which the aura is expanded but diffuse. In terms of energy, when the kundalini starts to rise, and we allow more energy to move through us, the auric field experiences an electromagnetic direct current or "DC" shift. The flow of electrons in the nervous system is increased and amplified to such a degree that all our internal processes are accelerated and expanded and we have access to thoughts, feelings and memories not accessible to us in our "normal" conscious state. In other words, this DC shift enables us to access our subconscious.

One of the advantages of a DC shift is that it enables us to feel more than one thing at a time. The problem is we usually cannot report those feelings. Most of the subjects who went through mystical or altered states in our studies had trouble reporting clearly.

[143] In the mid 1970's brain researchers at UCLA first discovered within the pineal gland a photochemical substance called melotonin. Later they found that melotonin is produced from serotonin, a neurotransmitter, also located in the pineal gland. They further discovered that stress caused an increase in the level of serotonin which in turn caused an increase in the production of melotonin. This increase plays a major role in creating a higher state of consciousness. The link between short-term stress and improved immunological response has also been scientifically recorded. (See Becker and Selden, op. cit.). It should be noted here, however, that while short-term stress has been shown to stimulate both one's immunological system and consciousness, continued stress seems to have the opposite effect. See Volume Six, for further discussion of the relation between stress, neurotransmitters and altered states.

It is my belief that the verbalization of the experience is hindered by language itself which is based upon reporting only one thing at a time. Consequently, culturally, language becomes a problem for us when we try to explain these kinds of experiences.

The most important part of the data we recorded at UCLA has now been incorporated by other scientists into an area called mind-field research. We alluded to this theory earlier in the book: that the mind is not simply situated in the brain, but, in fact, flows in, through and around the body. The DC shift not only makes available to us thoughts, feelings and memories previously locked within our subconscious, but this electromagnetic altered state also opens our minds to whatever is in the environment around us—words, images, emotions and so on. For this reason, the DC shift has also been described as "an open-mind field".[144] The significance of this is that each time we experience this shift in consciousness, each time we go into an altered state—whether it be as a result of meditation, hypnosis, trance, stress, illness or trauma—we are highly programmable.

Traumas and DC Shifts: Access to the Subconscious

Ordinarily trauma is the principle experience which brings on a DC shift. Most of us in fact have had the significant traumas of our lives recorded during a DC shift, which is why they are still in our subconscious and why they are still traumatic. We were "programmed". Since the DC shift is a way to access the subconscious mind, data that goes into the subconscious during a trauma

[144] Robert E. Ornstein, *The Mind Field*, New York: Pocket Books, 1976.

cannot be released from the subconscious until a shift of the same magnitude or intensity is again attained. As a result, though we might be able to recall the traumatic event, we cannot change any attitude we may have towards the experience (trauma). Neither can we alter how we feel or release the experience until we reach the amplitude of the original traumatic event again.

For example, the process of birth creates a DC shift in the baby. Therefore, we all have the potential to remember everything that went on during our birthing process, but usually do not. However, a person who is hypnotized (a process which creates an altered state) and taken back to his birth, will be able to report everything that happened during that experience.[145] To recall the data of a trauma consciously, one must somehow achieve that expanded field again. As our research revealed, physical therapies such as rolfing (as well as the energies transmitted in healing which also bring about a DC shift) are ways to reacquire this expanded field. Once this occurs, we are then able to change attitudes and feelings which, because they were linked to the traumatic experience, were also lodged within our subconscious. Because of their association with trauma and pain, these attitudes and feelings are often negative or destructive; at best they are restrictive. Locked within our subconscious, they continue to influence our thoughts and beliefs unconsciously. Once brought to consciousness, however, they can be examined, explored or simply released, making room for more healthy attitudes and feelings. Often during a rolfing or a healing session release will be sudden and accompanied by a flood of emotions.

[145] See Morris Netherton and Nancy Shiffrin, *Past Lives Therapy*, New York: William Morrow and Company, Inc., 1978.

Frequently, these emotions take the form of angry outbursts or tears, or a combination of both. Once these old angers and fears are surrendered, old patterns give way to newer and healthier ones.

Much of this was validated during our research. My own observations and personal experience have continued to support the findings and stimulate my interest in further research. The significance of the Rolf Study is perhaps best summed up by Valerie Hunt's concluding comments.

What do these detailed findings mean? The possible interpretations are staggering. These data constitute radiations taken directly from the body surface, quantitatively measured in a natural state containing frequencies and patterns that were isolated by scientifically accepted data reduction processes. Three different data resolutions by wave form, by Fourier frequency analysis and by a Sonogram frequency representation all produced the same results, differing only in the fineness of definition. Furthermore these findings taken from chakra locations were in direct correspondence with the aura reader's description of chakra energy and frequently depicted the total auric cloud. Throughout the centuries in which sensitives have seen and described the aura emissions, this is the first objective electronic evidence of frequency, amplitude and time, which validates their subjective observation of color discharge.

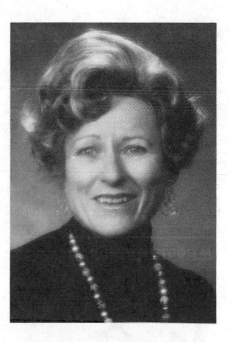

Fig. 5.5. DR. VALERIE V. HUNT.

...the extensive ram-
ifications for further study of
health, disease, pain, psychopathology and all human
behavior using the techniques
discovered in this study are
beyond estimation.[146]

The Meaning
of "Red" in American Culture

Although red is the color and energy of
the kundalini, and although our studies
found it to be very specifically related to an
awareness of life at the physical level, red is
not often associated with life or aliveness in
our culture. Instead, we relate it almost
exclusively to pain, accidents and traumas. It
is not an energy that we express or allow very
frequently. Perhaps we need to consider why
this is true.

In almost all cultures the appearance
of red in the aura is an indication of more
willingness to touch. We see this willingness
much more in several other societies.
Certainly it is true in Arab cultures; Arabic
people do touch more. It is also true
throughout the Mediterranean area of
Europe. However, it is not true for the
northern countries in Europe, from which
most of our Founding Fathers originated.
Most Americans tend to talk much more
about touch and sexuality than they actually
engage in either activity. This phenomenon
may also be related to considerations about
survival; when one's long-term survival is in
question, there is frequently more of a need to
seek comfort in the activities of touch and
sexuality which are associated with survival,
with life and with life-giving. Most of the

Arabic world is Third World, and the closer one gets to survival level, the more red appears in the aura. Most Arab people have magenta auras. As a collective group, Americans do not have the same considerations about survival as Third World cultures do. The further from that survival consciousness one moves, the less essential it seems to connect and reconnect with that life force.

Symbolically, our culture associates red with the command "stop!" Contrary to what our society teaches us, red does not mean "stop"; it means "go", "be alive". The cultural lesson in this ultimately is that as Americans we need to allow red to be more acceptable in our lives. Red carpeting is all right. Red clothing is all right. Healthy red blood is all right. Feeling alive is especially all right.

Chapter Six

DISEASE AND DYSFUNCTION

Sickle-Cell Anemia and Cancer: A Question of Power

In exploring the significance of red, there is a special need to discuss blood. Blood itself as a symbol is important. Blood is the red that runs appropriately throughout the body: it is the life force as the primitives knew it.[147] An all too common blood disease is anemia. Interestingly enough, in our culture women are described as having iron deficiency anemia because of their menstrual cycle. Anemia may be caused by lack of iron in a woman's diet, but it is more likely due to the lack of power that women have in our culture than to dietary deficiencies. Symbolically anemia represents lack of power.[148]

Iron deficiency anemia is not the only disease related to the issue of power. Sickle-cell anemia, and cancer, one of the more feared diseases of this era, are both related to the question of having, taking and using power appropriately. These diseases may thus be considered as being connected to the first chakra, since power originates in this center.

Sickle-cell anemia, which occurs

[147] This is why religions of antiquity incorporated various kinds of blood sacrifice. For example, the Goddess religions toward the last era of their practice (c. 2800-1800 B.C.) had an annual event in which the priestess chose a king every year, and at the end of the year he was let go—blood-let go. (See Sir James George Frazer, *The Golden Bough*, (one volume edition), New York: MacMillan Publishing Company, Inc., 1975, Chapter XXIV. This book is the classic and monumental [originally in 12 volumes, 1907-1915] survey of ancestral man's methods of worship, sex practices, magic, rituals and festivals.) According to Frazer, the ancient institution of divine kingship originated from the belief that the well-being of nature and society depended upon the vitality of the king, who must therefore be slain when his powers began to fail him. He would then be replaced by a healthier successor. There was obviously much injustice around that. Although the development of patriarchal societies is a broad subject whose discussion is beyond the scope of this book, I believe that the patriarchy arose in part because of the injustice of the matristic societies which preceded them. (The terms *patriarchy* and *matriarchy* have fallen into disuse among most anthropologists and ethnologists. I use the terms here not to denote either male or female dominated societies but rather to refer to cultures and epochs in which either the worship of the Goddess or of the male Deity predominated.) I do not think, however, that patriarchy was a cycle that arose simply as a result of rebellion. At the time there was much of a transformed kind of vibration occurring, so more than likely it arose primarily as a part of the natural evolutionary cycle. Certainly as the focus of society changed from the basic hunting-gathering culture of the neolithic age to the agrarian-village cultures and finally expanded into a civilization of city-states, so too was the form of worship bound to change. (For further discussion of this process, refer to Campbell, *The Masks of God: Oriental Mythology*, op. cit.) For another point of view on this topic, see Gerda Lerner, *The Origins of Patriarchy*.

[148] It is beyond the scope of this book to present a complete discussion of the symbology of diseases. The subject will be thoroughly treated in an upcoming book by me which is presently in progress. However, as a disease or its symbology relates to the functioning or dysfunctioning of a particular chakra, it will be noted and herein briefly discussed.

213

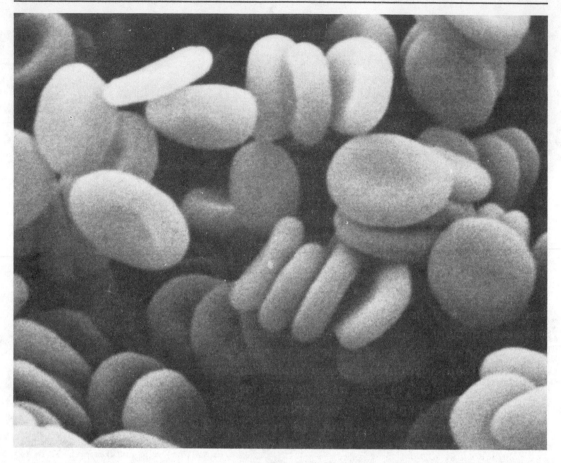

Fig. 6.1. Shown above: NORMAL RED BLOOD CELLS
Enlarged 10,000 times. Omikron/Photo Researchers, Inc.

Fig. 6.2. NORMAL RED BLOOD CELLS COMPARED TO
SICKEL CELLED BLOOD. Dr. Tony Brain/Science Photo
Library/Photo Researchers, Inc.

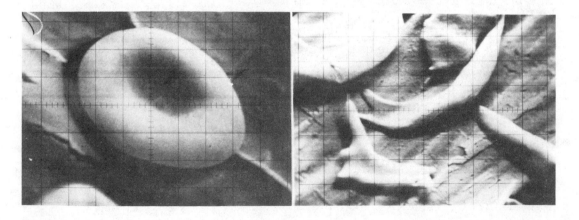

mainly in the Black race, is caused by an abnormal hemoglobin (hemoglobin SS, or Hb SS), which is sensitive to oxygen deficiency. When oxygen is reduced, the result is distorted and elongated red blood cells, which eventually become rigid and sickle-shaped. Ultimately this sickling leads to irreversible distortion of the cells, resulting in obstruction of blood circulation and the eventual fragmentation of the red cells. One might say it is as though the cell "explodes". On a symbolic level, this "explosion" occurs because the power associated with a particular way of being is repressed. Instead of being expressed or having an environment in which to be expressed, it gets stuck in the body and eventually causes death. A wonderful life force, instead of being developed and used, is smothered. Once our culture as a whole is no longer threatened by a powerful life force, it will be interesting to see whether the occurrence of these blood diseases diminishes.

Cancer, perhaps more than any other disease, represents a misuse of power. Whenever there is a cell that runs amok, as it does in cancer, a power problem is indicated. In cancer the body believes that the tumor which has been created should be protected and attended to in the same way as an injury, so it sends its blood supply to the tumor and feeds it. The body uses the wrong kind of power for the wrong thing in the wrong place. It thinks it is repairing the cell when in fact it is nurturing the deadly tumor. The body sends in red blood cells when what it needs to fight a tumor are white blood cells.

As a general rule, cancer patients often consider themselves to be undeserving. Their lives are filled with crises and loss.[149] They have difficulty accepting and using power

[149] Cancer and the cancer patient are also discussed in Volume II. For more on the psychological profile of cancer patients, see Becker and Selden, op. cit., pp. 221-225.

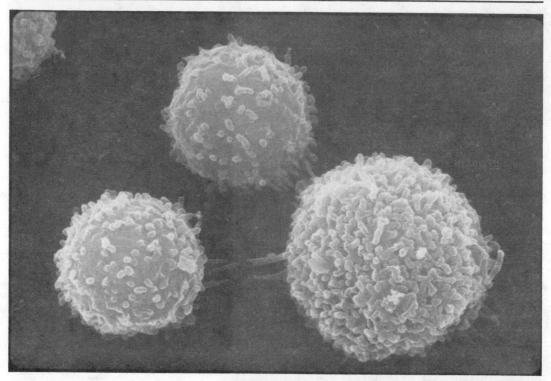

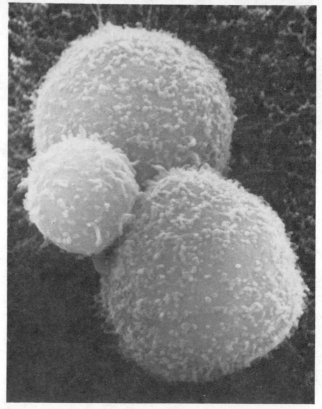

Fig. 6.3. LYMPHOCYTES. B and T Cells. (Scanning Electron Microscope Photograph). Don Fawcett/Science Source/Photo Researchers, Inc.

Fig. 6.4. T-LYMPHOCYTE. Immune T-Lymphocyte (small cell) attacks two large tumour cells. (Scanning Electron Microscope Photograph). Dr. A. Liepins/Science Photo Library/Photo Researchers, Inc.

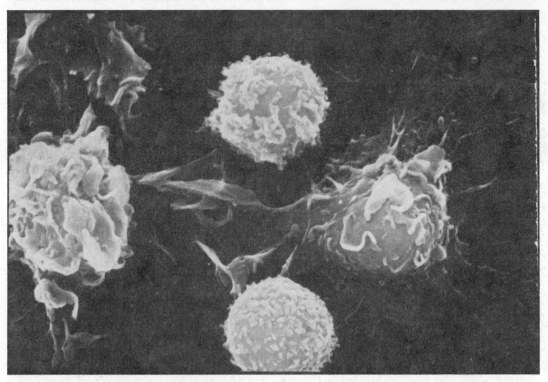

Fig. 6.5. CANCER CELLS (to left and right). Dividing lymphocytes seen at top and bottom. SEM. Nina Lampen/Science Source/Photo Researchers, Inc.

properly. Lack of vitality in the first chakra, lack of orange frequency in the second chakra, inappropriate use of power, as well as grief and fear are connected to the body's inability to produce white blood cells to fight off malignancy. When cancer patients reorder their psychological inventories, their bodies can and will fight the disease.

The Cancer Cell

A cancerous cell is a low frequency, low amplitude embryonic cell. This means that the cell, instead of vibrating at the same rate as the body, vibrates at a much slower energy or frequency—the same frequency, in fact, as that of embryonic cells.[150] When a cell slows its vibration, the body thinks it is making a baby and consequently allows that

[150] Becker and Selden, op. cit.

217

cell to multiply and divide rapidly, which is what causes the tumorous growth. Then it sends in blood supply to feed those cells; most tumors, if they are not being treated, grow at the same rate as a baby grows. Thus, an appropriate treatment, and one which has been done in research settings,[151] is to raise the frequency of the malignant cell. In the research environment, an electrode is attached to the cancerous area and then an electrical current vibrating at the base frequency of the body (about 8-1/2 cycles per second) is introduced. Although this does not really reduce the tumor, it does change the cells: the cells stop being embryonic and start being the same kind of cells as the ones adjacent to them.[152] This is similar to what happens in a healing process. Take for example a breast mass. To a healer a breast tumor feels as if it is melting under his hands. It is not actually melting; it has begun to dedifferentiate. Transformation at a cellular level is the healer's goal.

Cancer Treatment

The basic healing treatment for cancer patients begins with work to open the feeder systems—the parts of the body that feed it energy on a continuous basis. Next we must check to see if the chakras are balanced, then work on the organ that is damaged or on the tumor, wherever it might be. Finally, we must seal off the field so that the client can continue to regenerate energy and not lose it so easily.

When we discuss the feeder system of the body, we are referring primarily to the feet and knees, the hips, the shoulders and the hands. We live in a force field, and our feet and knees are the first two places that energy

[151] Ibid.

[152] Ibid.

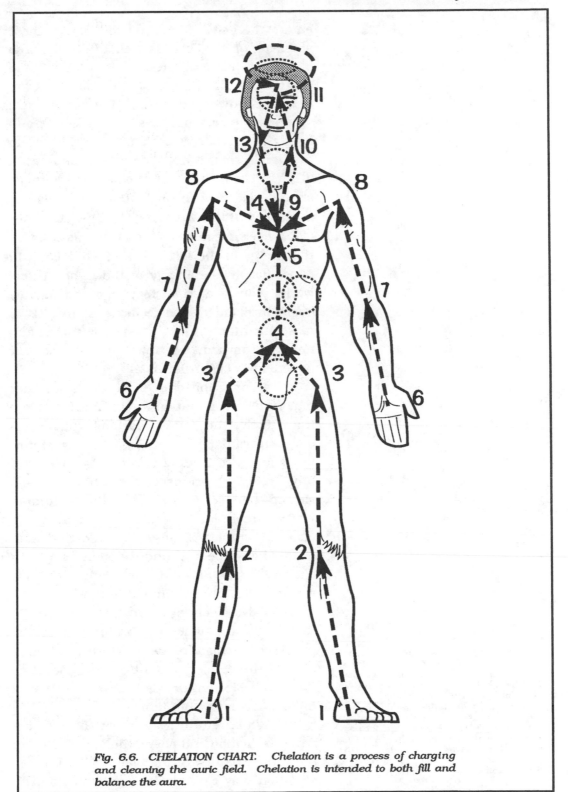

Fig. 6.6. CHELATION CHART. *Chelation is a process of charging and cleaning the auric field. Chelation is intended to both fill and balance the aura.*

enters the body. We need to know if these areas are open. There is a chakra in the arch of the foot just as there is one in the palm of the hand. The hips and the shoulders are primary power centers. The knees are secondary power sources, and the feet and hands are tertiary chakras. The chakras in the hands spin in opposite directions to each other. The energy of the feet and knees should also flow in opposition. It does not matter which way the energy moves—clockwise or counter-clockwise—as long as the energy of the left foot and knee flows in opposition to the energy of the right. If one works palm chakra to foot, one can usually begin to open up the feeder systems. It is most important to keep these flows open and moving upward, particularly with cancer patients but ideally for us all.

In treating cancer, there is another important consideration for the healer. More than likely, the cancer patient will be undergoing radiation or chemotherapy simultaneously with healing treatments, or he will have recently undergone such therapies. Healers must clear out all of the pollutants which are the side effects of these other cancer therapies. The way we do that is to channel into the liver and the kidneys and *to chelate*[153] (see Fig. 6.6) the client each time we see him. In other words, we treat the whole body: channel energy from the feet to the head and balance the brain. The higher purple and indigo frequencies are effective in raising the cancer patient's energy level so that his basic vibration is higher than that of the malignancy within him.

While retarding the growth of malignancy, radiation and chemotherapy also lower the basic vibration of the body. That lowered vibration may cause more malignant growth

[153] *Chelation* is a process of charging and clearing the aura. To "chelate" is derived from the Greek *chele* which means "claw". In the chelation process, energy is channeled into the client's body in progressive steps beginning at the feet and moving up the body and the chakra system. Since energy is usually drawn into the body from the earth through the feet, this process brings energy into the body in the most natural way. Chelation is intended to both fill and balance the aura.

later on.[154] Often a new tumor will appear as a result of radiation eighteen months from the date of the last radiation treatment.[155] With radiation or chemotherapy, the new group of cells which is growing does not get enough energy, so again cancerous cells are produced. Thus, we have to raise the energy level of the whole unit. We have to keep the energy high enough long enough to produce a whole new set of healthy cells. Therefore, cancer patients must be treated immediately following their "spontaneous remission".

What usually happens, however, is that the cancer patient is overjoyed at the "remission", comes back to the healer, and says, "I'm well, and I'm not coming back for any more treatment." At this point, the healer on the case should say, "What a minute; I don't think I'm willing to participate in your decision not to continue treatment." This is not the time for the healer to jump to conclusions and pat himself on the back. The cancer patient has just been clutched from death's grasp, and he must learn to live again. If he is insistent on stopping treatment, the healer needs to explain the possible effects of radiation. It is essential to clean out radiation and chemicals in order for the cancer patient to continue to live in true health. Furthermore, continued treatment is necessary to support the cancer patient in his new approach to life.

Arthritis, Colitis and Alzheimer's Disease

There are several other diseases associated with the first chakra. Among them is Alzheimer's disease. It is estimated that in the U.S. two to three million people are

[154] Refer to *The Merck Manual of Diagnosis and Therapy*, op. cit., pp. 1729-1734.

[155] See Helen Caldicott, *Nuclear Madness*, New York: Bantam, 1981, and Becker and Selden, op. cit., pp. 218-219.

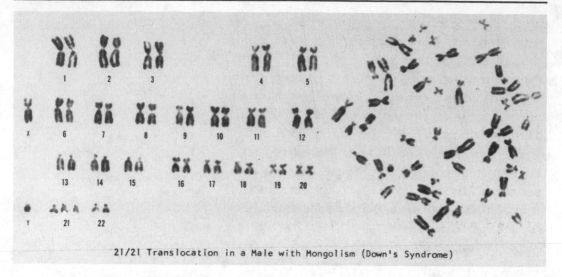

21/21 Translocation in a Male with Mongolism (Down's Syndrome)

Fig. 6.7. CELLULAR ABNORMALITY IN DOWN'S SYNDROME. 21/21 Translocation in Male with Down's Syndrome (Mongolism). Leonard Lessin/ Photo Researchers, Inc.

affected by Alzheimer's,[156] a disease evidenced by a slow, continuous decline in intellectual function. At first the medical profession thought Alzheimer's was senility, or the cause of senile dementia. Lately, however, Alzheimer's has come to be recognized as the major cause of mental deterioration in both the elderly and the middle-aged. Research has revealed that individuals affected by Alzheimer's have a diminished level of neurotransmitters, critical brain molecules that are essential for the communication of brain cells. Thus far, however, the cause of Alzheimer's remains a mystery. Theories range from environmental aluminum toxicity or viral infection to genetic abnormality or premature aging of the brain. Interestingly, Alzheimer's has recently been linked with Down's syndrome, a disorder originating with the inception of life: two recent studies revealed symptoms of Alzheimer's disease in about 25% of adult Down's syndrome patients.[157] Even more significant, when brains of adults with Down's syndrome are microscopically examined, tissue often shows cellular abnormalities

[156] Edward L. Schneider, M.D., "Aging", *Encyclopaedia Britannica, Medical and Health Annual*, 1987, p. 271.

[157] Ibid., p. 400.

apparently identical to those seen in the brains of victims of Alzheimer's. These abnormal structures—neuritic plaques and neurofibrillary tangles—appear to be the result of degeneration of nerve cells.[158] Eventual confusion, disorientation and severe memory loss characterize Alzheimer's. This last characteristic—complete loss of memory— makes it apparent that kundalini flow has stopped altogether, since it is the kundalini which allows the flow of energy to access information and bring it to the conscious level. A healer friend of mine used to say that a healer treats Alzheimer's "from crotch to crown". This is truly good advice for treating diseases that affect the entire consciousness, and certainly Alzheimer's is one of those diseases.

Arthritis is another dysfunction of the first chakra. The arthritic has diverted his life force—his red energy—to the joints. The body's initial message to send red to the joints is a result of the individual's inability to express or experience his anger. Once the red gets to the joints and starts causing pain, the patient resists the pain which becomes even more severe because of the resistance. Arthritis may be considered a "resistance" disease: the arthritic first resists any expression of anger and then resists the pain of the inflammation (the anger) within the joints. A healer best treats arthritis with alternating red and white frequencies. With rheumatoid arthritis, one has to first remove the inflammation from the joint, which requires green and blue to transform the red (inflammatory) frequency. Once this is accomplished, the healer then has to rebuild the joints, which requires the regenerative red frequency be restored appropriately.

Like arthritis, colitis is an inflam-

[158] Ibid.

matory disease. While the arthritic has attempted to avoid his anger, the colitis patient attempts to avoid all feelings. The colitis patient always has a second chakra that runs backwards. He has stopped the information loop by turning his second chakra around. If for some reason a person does not want a piece of information or stimulus to move up the system, if he does not like the way it feels, he will turn a chakra in the opposite direction so that the information loop cannot be completed. A colitis patient turns his second chakra the wrong way so that all the life force that comes up the system hits his emotional body and goes right back down causing increased peristaltic action or "dumping syndrome". Emotions never reach an area where they can be expressed.

I have never treated colitis or diverticulitis in which the second chakra is not backwards, causing dysfunction in the first chakra, thus making the intestine inflamed. Inflamed means full of red; instead of the red being where it belongs, it is all over, thereby continually recirculating the inflammation. The whole intestine is lacerated. If the client allowed himself one honest feeling, it would turn the chakra the right way, and healing could begin.

Inflammatory Disease: Anger, Fear and Pain

Most inflammatory diseases, no matter where they are localized in the body, are usually related indirectly to anger or fear and most certainly are related in a more direct way to pain. As already noted, this is especially true of arthritis and colitis. While anger, fear and pain are in themselves natural ways for the body to protect itself, misdirected or suppressed anger, repressed or excessive fear and chronic pain are all indications of imbalance in the first chakra.

Remember that anger in its pure state is often a starter for the body but is frequently expressed as violence. Therefore people often suppress anger because they are afraid of the possible violent outcome or because they do not trust their process, or both. However, when anger is suppressed for these reasons, one has denied the processing that the body—the chakra system—is capable of doing. If we can learn to stop repressing the anger and start trusting that the body knows how to handle it, we realize what a beautiful and effective system we have. Anger comes up, becomes a feeling, becomes an opinion and becomes a second feeling. It is when any part of that process or system is circumvented that the danger exists anger will be expressed as violence or that we might actually hurt somebody.

Fear resides in both the first and second centers, depending on whether we are feeling our own fear or whether we are being affected by another's fear. If for instance, I am afraid in and of myself, my fear is going to draw from the first center; I am going to feel it at the base of the spine. On the other hand, if you are afraid and your fear affects me, I am first going to become aware of it in my second center.

While our own fear tends to be centered in the first chakra, if we are afraid for another, that fear may tend to move from our second chakra into our first as well. In other words, the body will tend to *sense* all fear in the first chakra. If the source of the fear is outside of ourselves, then we need to consider its potential damage factor to determine if it is life-threatening. If the problem is life-threatening, fear should register in the first chakra so that we can take the proper action to ensure the survival of the life force.

Fear of life and of feeling often drive people into chronic pain. Pain patients displace all of their red energy—anger, rage, fear, passion—in order to avoid feeling alive. In many cases, if sexuality is added to their relationships, it increases their suffering. They will take that extra input of red and run it directly into the pain, which consequently increases.

A person in pain is isolating himself: in order to stay in that painful state, one has to maintain red outside the first chakra for a long time. Transforming this pattern is especially difficult because the power necessary for this transformation has been displaced with the red.

Consequently, there are some important considerations for healers who treat clients with chronic pain. If red frequency is channeled into a client who is in pain, he will displace this energy into his pain and thus feel pain more pronouncedly. Therefore, red is not the frequency of choice for a pain patient, at least not until much of the pain has been pulled out and eased. A "cooler" frequency such as green or blue should be chosen. Secondly, when a body is using a particular energy inappropriately, a healer can help the client redirect that energy; for example, the energy in an inflamed joint can be better used to make red blood cells. Removing red or inflammation from the body, does not deprive the first chakra of red energy. We are not short circuiting the client.

Red energy, flowing appropriately,

does the same thing in all bodies. If we bring up the life force vigorously, whether it is through jogging, sit-ups or channeling energy, we get sore muscles, we get hot and cold flashes in the body, or what feels like a rush of warm water, and tingling dilation of the capillaries. We get many funny little sensations, which are only indications that our body is growing or changing to carry the energy. Healers' bodies change dramatically the longer and more intensely they channel energy; they acquire the wiring to run ever higher frequencies. What happens at first, and the reason they feel sensations, is that they are feeling the resistance to a higher energy than they have run before. In other words, they are running 220 volts, and they are only wired for 110. Thus, as the body tries to rewire itself, there will be symptoms, but that is all they are and they should not be given much attention other than to notice something is happening.

Hypertension and Heart Disease

Like cancer, heart disease is a result of the inappropriate use of red energy. Heart disease, and its risk factor, high blood pressure or hypertension, can be considered a major disease of the first chakra.

High blood pressure is often one of the first signs of heart disease. Like arthritis, high blood pressure is a result of misdirected anger. Whereas the arthritic has displaced his red energy to the joint, the hypertensive has displaced all his anger to his head. Aurically, the hypertensive, instead of having a crown chakra, will have two yellow plumes spouting off the two acupuncture points at

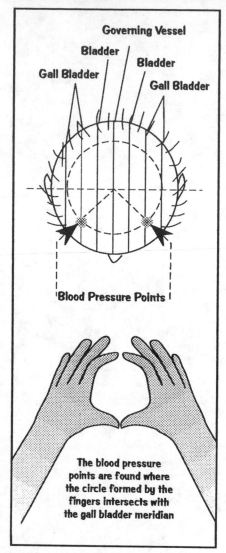

Governing Vessel

Bladder

Bladder

Gall Bladder

Gall Bladder

Blood Pressure Points

The blood pressure points are found where the circle formed by the fingers intersects with the gall bladder meridian

Fig. 6.8. BLOOD PRESSURE MERIDIANS. Two meridian points on the head are especially good for treating high blood pressure. Computer drawing by M.M. Smith/Techni-Visions.

the top of the crown. To treat hypertension, the healer needs to run the energy down the body, directing red energy back into the first chakra. If the client is on blood pressure medication, this is especially important to do. Such medications are designed to limit the body's response to stimuli and often diminish sexual function. The healer needs to put the red energy and the anger back where they belong, in the first chakra, so the patient feels alive again and before the anger literally kills someone, namely the patient himself.

Next, the healer should balance the chakras one at a time. In other words, he needs to channel red frequency into the first chakra, orange into the second, yellow into the third, green into the fourth, blue into the fifth, violet into the sixth and white into the crown and then make certain that the colors are stable in each chakra. If the healer can get the hypertensive to visualize the appropriate colors through a meditation, the process is facilitated.

Similar to the arthritic, the hypertensive usually starts his disease with a pattern of repressed hostility. When we consider that heart disease is the number one killer in our country, we are forced also to consider our society's attitude toward anger. In our culture it is difficult to find an appropriate outlet for anger. Sexuality can often be expressed in subtle ways, but this is not the case with anger. And when anger and hostility are misdirected and find expression in sexuality, serious social problems result. As a culture we have not yet acknowledged that power can be expressed sexually, actively, creatively, emotionally, in anger and in passion. There are many ways to express fire.

Genetic Disease

Because the first chakra holds the energy of life itself, which is responsible for the creation of the physical body, genetic disease must be considered a disease of the first chakra. Any disease that is genetically carried is being rapidly proliferated at this time on the planet. I tend to think that this phenomenon is post-Hiroshima. It is quite apparent that the world as we know it today is not anything like the pre-war world. Since we discovered that we can split the atom, which was thought to be impossible, there have also been "atomic" kinds of explosions in consciousness.

The awesome possibility of total annihilation dwarfs the individual's sense of himself as being capable and powerful enough to affect his own survival. Such anxiety and confusion reverberates at a cellular level. The Atomic Age, in exploding our concept of reality, has brought our very cellular integrity into question. Tay-Sachs, sickle cell anemia, cancer and AIDS are all diseases that are cellular in nature and in which the integrity of the cell or the unit has been jeopardized.

I am sorry to report that the treatment of genetic disease seems to be the one major area in which healing has been the least effective. While some cellular diseases such as cancer have responded to healing, genetic disease per se has not. We may as a planet need to change the way we use energy before we can become more effective in this area. One thing is for certain. Before the proliferation of genetic disease becomes the norm for our society, we must not only discover a more creative way to deal with atomic energy, but we must also find within ourselves the integrity to redirect our own fragmented energy, to harness our own power.

Bacterial and Viral Infections, Broken Bones and Scar Tissue: Healing With Red Frequency

Genetic disease, cancer, arthritis and Alzheimer's are all serious illnesses associated with the first chakra and with the imbalance of first chakra energies. However, there are less serious medical problems which, because they are treated with the red frequency of the first chakra, are also connected to this first center and need to be discussed.

There is probably no one who has not had an infection of some kind, either bacterial or viral. Bacteria exists in the lower red harmonic. However, it is a very strong frequency, which is why a bacterial infection rips through the body so quickly. Interestingly, channeling a lot of red energy actually gets rid of bacteria, for it forces the bacteria into the next higher harmonic of red, a harmonic in which it can no longer thrive.

Broken bones are also healed with red frequency. Actually, I use red and white alternating frequencies. The white frequency causes liquefaction of the bone edges and the red regenerates the bone tissue, both of which are needed to prevent later scarring in a broken bone. Scarring tends to build up frequency resistance later on, so it should be avoided if at all possible.

Wherever there are cut cells in the body, neuroblast, fibroblast and osteoblast patch and repair systems are found. We have recently seen scientific documentation for what healers knew a long time ago: that those cells, because they were cut through, and because there were too many extra cells, did not get enough energy to them to form perfectly.[159] Thus scar tissue is a retarded cell and that is what makes up its thick consistency and its insulative quality. To treat it, we need to blast it with enough powerful red energy to turn it back into a more normal cell. In general, whenever we need to "burn" anything out of the body, or whenever any kind of regeneration is indicated, the powerful red frequency of the first chakra is the frequency of choice.

Treating Overdoses

Since addictions are associated with repressed kundalini, drug overdose, while it is not a disease per se, can certainly cause a dysfunction of the first center. When someone is lying face down on the ground somewhere, we do not have much time to think about what we are going to do. First aid is certainly the first and most appropriate course of treatment, and a word of caution is needed here. Shock can result from major overdoses of most drugs. A person in shock as a result of overdose is in a critical condition. Elimination of the drug in such an individual is contingent upon first restoring blood pressure to a safe level. Then the level of the drug in the bloodstream must be changed as quickly as possible. As a healer, the fastest way to do that is to channel energy into the liver and kidneys to flush them out. Red is the frequency to channel for most overdoses.

Cocaine, which has become the most abused drug next to alcohol, turns the whole auric field silver, a color associated with the high frequency of the eighth chakra, the

[159] Becker and Selden, op. cit.

231

Atman, which is connected to divine power. This is why users often think they are so invulnerable. Again, a red frequency will flush the metal and transform the silver to a more "down-to-earth" vibration.

Gynecological Problems and the Effects of the Hysterectomy

Our culture especially has far too many gynecological problems. Women need to have an open kundalini in order to avoid such problems. While some women who are able to deliver babies easily are relatively open in the first center, the majority of American women are plagued with problems in this area. These problems extend from irregular menstrual cycles to chronic vaginitis to being pre-orgasmic. All such problems are indicative of a closed first chakra and of women not giving themselves permission to be open inside: they give themselves no permission to be in touch with their own fire energy. There is a fear there, a fear of their own power. Sometimes the kinds of things that would make a woman afraid are loss of love, loss of a job, loss of an education or loss of a relationship. It is the loss of whatever makes one feel alive that could lead a person to close off the first chakra.

In general, healers should treat most sexual dysfunctions with both red and green frequencies. Green is the power behind red. The problem behind most sexual dysfunctions is trust or lack of it. Trust is a quality which resides in the heart center. In other words, lack of heart chakra is one major cause of sexual dysfunctions. Lack of openness, lack of embrace, some of the qualities which are associated with the heart center, affect the kundalini. Thus, often a sexually dysfunctional first chakra must be treated with both red and green frequencies.

In this culture, medicine's answer to a woman who has had a history of gynecological problems is for her to have a hysterectomy. A hysterectomy has a very damaging effect on the energy flow of the first chakra. A hysterectomy cuts three meridians, and in doing so seriously harms the first chakra's ability to produce red, life force itself.

What this means to a woman who has had a hysterectomy is that she must reconnect her meridians energetically; she must keep that chakra running. Her body will be healthy and full of vitality as long as her first chakra energy is consistent. Sometimes the meridians will reconnect naturally. When this does not occur, the healer should channel red frequency to bring about the desired reconnection.

After a woman has had a hysterectomy, or during menopause, what is prescribed for her is a hormone, estrogen, to replace the hormone that was produced formerly by her ovaries. Estrogen is also produced to a small extent in the adrenals. If the ovaries continue producing estrogen, a woman's skin stays young looking. In fact, aging is slowed because that hormone, estrogen, is the frequency modulator for the red vibration in the entire field. Anywhere there is an even balance of red, each skin cell that reproduces, reproduces perfectly, as the one before. The quantity of estrogen, then, is not the important factor; it is the steadiness of the estrogen level, the consistency with which that vibration is produced that keeps us vital and young. The point is, it is not important to have estrogen, but it is very important to have red consistently and completely all the time.

It just happens that estrogen is the modulator for this very necessary frequency.

Opportunistic Viruses and Infections: Treating Sexually Transmitted Diseases

As far as diseases of the first chakra go, sexually transmitted diseases are probably at the top of the list. In our society perhaps the most prolific sexual disease which affects both men and women is herpes. In treating herpes, as in cancer treatment, healers need to change cellular structure. Some medical practitioners and researchers in fact believe that herpes, like other viruses, may be a forerunner to certain forms of cancer. It is a virus, it moves and proliferates very rapidly, and it is highly contagious. Unlike bacteria, a microorganism which lives off the body and the body's strength, a virus is so minute in size that it can reside and proliferate within a single living cell (the *host* cell). From this hiding place it gains strength and number and can move in any direction to colonize other cells.

Once in the body a virus may have an unapparent effect, living dormantly in the host cell. It may destroy the cell but cause it to divide before it dies, thereby proliferating the virus. It may also transform the cell, causing it to take on abnormal growth patterns and become cancerous. Some viruses produce latent infections, persisting in a quiescent state and becoming periodically active in acute episodes. Such is the case with herpes.

Whereas a bacterial infection indicates the need to change how we *feel* (usually with regard to anger), a viral infection indicates the need to change how we *think*, not our opinions, but a "wholesale change" in consciousness.

Many of the more recent sexually transmitted diseases (STD's) are viral because much of our generation has been mating without expressing the full vitality and passion of the root chakra. We have split off some important parts of our power and have withheld the life force from self and other. This lack of fire creates the environment for a virus, which lives in a higher, "cooler" frequency than a bacteria, to take hold.

In treating the viral STD's, such as herpes and AIDS, the ethics, attitudes and consciousness around the position that sexuality and power hold in one's life must be addressed. Obviously the time for casual encounters is over. One change in consciousness that must emerge from these viruses is the awareness that sexual union is the sacred joining of two life forces. We must begin to be more selective about the kind and quality of energy with which we choose to merge.

Bacteria tend to be inflammatory because they live within the slower, "hotter" harmonics of red-orange. They, unlike the virus, cannot grow in the higher, faster, "cooler" frequencies. Therefore, the healer needs to channel "cool" energy, such as blue and green, to inhibit their growth.

In treating viruses, it has been my experience that the red-purple frequencies are the most effective; the purple calls forth the soul to intervene in effecting the needed changes in consciousness, while the red rebuilds the life force itself. In a sense, the healer must seek not only to "burn out" the virus but also to "burn away" aspects of the client's consciousness which interfere with his

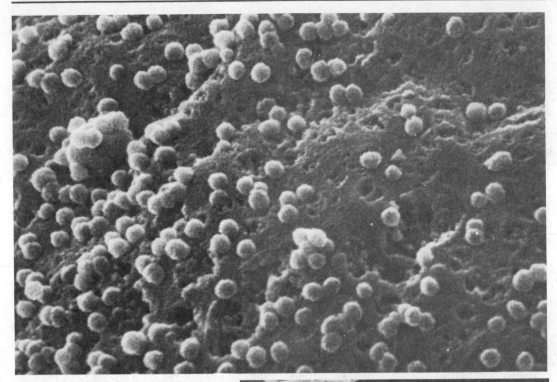

Fig. 6.9. Above: AIDS VIRUS. Enlarged 50,000 times. SEM. Cecil Fox/NIH/Science Source/Photo Researchers,Inc..

Fig. 6.10. Right: HTLV-3. Infected T-4 lymphocytes shows virus budding from plasma membrane. CDC/Science Source/Photo Researchers, Inc.

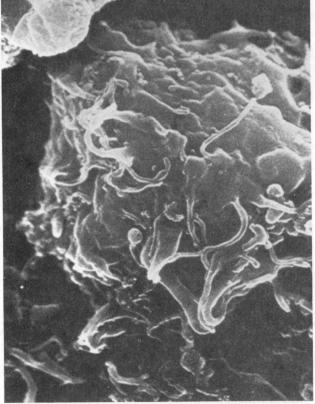

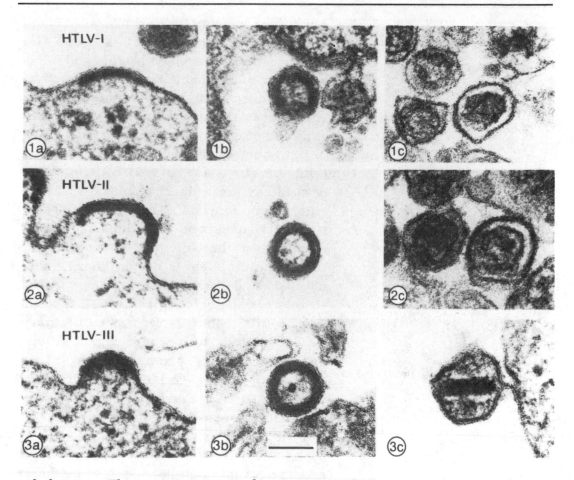

Fig. 6.11. Above: HTLV I, II, III. AIDS VIRUS. Dr. Robert Gallo/NCI/Photo Researchers, Inc.

wholeness. The consciousness of a virus is an interplay of thought (how we think) and life force (how we live). These often fragmented or opposing aspects of ourselves must be brought into balance. *Wholeness* means *wholesomeness*: recognizing and surrounding ourselves with those people and things which bring light and life while also being able to identify "the enemy"—that which takes away light and life. We must learn to protect ourselves from that which can harm us. We must learn to use anger and sexuality in ways which clear the body, promote growth and increase vitality and life force. It is already too much that this generation feels unsafe with the impersonal dark cloud of nuclear devastation hanging over our heads. Without the ability to choose what is "good" for us—that which is safe and healthy and full of light—our autoimmune systems cannot and will not protect us from the onslaught—and in some cases the annihilation—of rampant virus and disease.

Some of the more serious diseases (and in the case of AIDS, the more devastating) are a direct result of weakened autoimmune function. These are the *opportunistic* viruses and infections, so called because every time the body is depleted and the immune system is not on guard, these infections and diseases seize the "opportunity" to overtake the "compromised" system. Besides AIDS, which by its very nature must be considered the premier opportunistic disease, two other "opportunists" which have been getting a great deal of attention recently are *Candidiasis*, or *Candida*, which is actually a systemic fungal disease, and the *Epstein-Barr* virus (EBV).

Candidiasis is often referred to simply as a "yeast" infection because it is produced by the yeastlike fungus *Candida Albicans*, a common inhabitant of the mouth, vagina and intestinal tract. Prolonged treatment with broad-spectrum antibiotics (mainly the tetracyclines) seems to predispose one to developing candidiasis, since such treatment tends to kill off the body's normal bacterial antagonists to the fungus.

Although candida can infect several areas of the body, it is most commonly characterized by intermittent inflammation of the bowel and vagina. Perhaps the greatest difficulty with candida is coping with the allergic reactions it causes. The body often becomes hypersensitive to things to which it was never sensitive before.

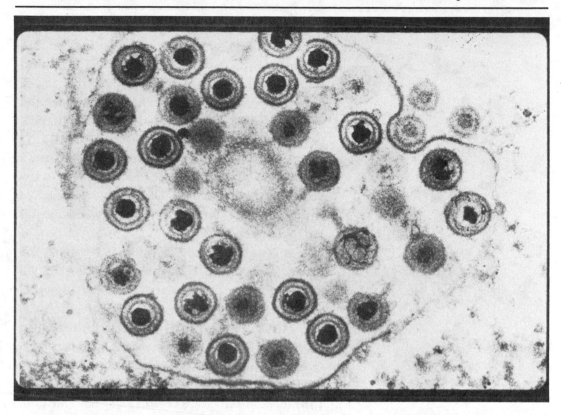

Nystatin, an antifungal antibiotic, is often prescribed for one infected with candida; eliminating such things as dairy products, sugars and yeast-based or fermented foods from one's diet is also recommended in most cases. Candidiasis becomes active and thrives in hotter, moist environments. Therefore, from a healing perspective, the higher ("cooler") frequencies of energy are most effective in treating it. From any perspective, however, candidiasis is difficult to treat, for, as with all the "opportunistic" infections, the body's best defense mechanism—the immune system—has been compromised.

The Epstein-Barr virus (EBV) is the fifth and most recently described herpesvirus (see Table Fig. 6.13)[160] and like all other herpesviruses, EBV is latent, persisting in the

Fig. 6.12. HERPES SIMPLEX VIRUS. CDC/Science Source/Photo Researchers, Inc.

[160] See Stephen E. Straus, M.D., "The Epstein-Barr Virus", *Medical and Health Annual, Encyclopaedia Britannica*, 1987, pp. 471, 473.

body for life. In addition to being associated with acute infectious mononucleosis, the Epstein-Barr virus (EBV) has also been related to Burkett's lymphoma, a rare form of lymphoid cancer characterized by unchecked growth of EBV- transformed white blood cells, B lymphocytes.[161] The presence of EBV in the saliva or of infected cells in one's bloodstream is not indicative of the disease, however, and lifetime carriage of Epstein-Barr virus seems inconsequential for most people.[162]

Epstein-Barr has been termed the "yuppy" disease by some because of its prevalence among young, usually well-educated and fairly affluent professionals. The virus, like many of those it infects, also tends to "live well" in a weakened system. One infected with EBV may have symptoms similar to those of mononucleosis—fever, sore throat, swollen glands and extreme fatigue. Fatigue is the most characteristic symptom. The body is simply exhausted. But most people ignore all the exhaustion signals. On some level it is as if an intellectual superiority prevents one from believing he could have a weakened immune system. The situation is complicated even further when we consider another factor specific to EBV. Not only does the viral nature of Epstein-Barr make it difficult to treat, but this specific virus is not unique to any one location in the body. It attacks whichever nerve seems to be weakest within its host. This means that not only can EBV manifest differently in different people; it may even manifest in various locations over a period of time within the same individual.

The more we understand about the nature of viruses and the more we see how different viruses function in the body, the more apparent it becomes that the discoveries

---

[161] Ibid., p. 473.

[162] Ibid.

VIRUS	Usual Age of Infection	% Infected by Age 40	Major Associated Diseases
Herpes Simples 1	Childhood	50-70	Herpes sores of the mouth, eyes or skin
Herpes Simplex 2	Adolescence to Adult	20-50	Herpes sores of genitals and adjacent skin
Varicella-Zoster	Childhood	80-90	Chicken Pox, Shingles
Cytomegalovirus	All	50-70	Hepatitis, Mononucleosis, congenital infections
Epstein Barr	Childhood to Adolescence	80-100	Infections, Mononucleosis

Fig. 6.13. EPSTEIN-BARR VIRUS. Relation between Epstein-Barr virus and other human herpes viruses. Britannica Medical and Health Annual, 1987, p.472.

being made about viruses within this and the next generations will revolutionize our knowledge of the body in the same way that discoveries about bacteria did in the last century. Although bacteria and virus are both living organisms, bacteria may live in any environment—soil, water, air and organic matter, as well as in the bodies of plants and animals. On the other hand, once outside of a living cell, a virus is much more likely to become a lifeless particle. Nevertheless, a viral infection is much more difficult to treat than a bacterial one. A major factor which makes treatment of the virus so much more difficult is that while both bacteria and viruses are microscopic, a bacterium is a single-celled organism, but a virus is so small that it lives and grows *within* a single-cell. By

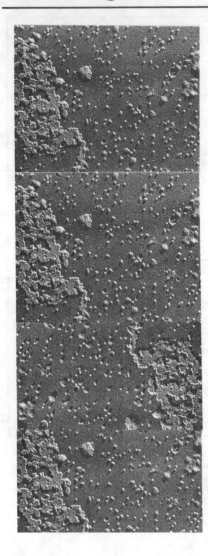

Fig. 6.14. Left: POLIO VIRUS. Omikron/ Photo Researchers, Inc.

Fig. 6.15. Top right: BACTERIA. Comparing Fig. 6.14 with Fig. 6.15, we can more easily understand the difficulty in treating a virus, which is so minute in size that it can live within the single-celled bacterium. Dr. Tony Brain/ Science Photo Library/Photo Researchers, Inc.

Fig. 6.16. Bottom right: THE CELL. The cell consists of several structures. Shown here is the cell's nucleus, the control center where the blueprints for cellular activity originate. From the nucleus, the genetic material passes out into the surrounding cytoplasm by means of several pores in the membrane. The dark stained area around the inner periphery, and scattered within the nucleus, is chromatin—the unorganised form the chromosomes take in a cell that is not undergoing cell division. The gray area surrounding the nucleus is the cytoplasm, which is full of tiny bodies each responding to instructions from the nucleus. The black-dotted squiggles are strands of endoplasmic reticulum containing ribosomes. Protein synthesis for the cell occurs here. Many of the light gray sausage-like shapes and some of the oval bodies are mitochondria, which release energy, thereby enabling the cell to grow and divide. Dr. Brian Eyden/Science Photo Library/Photo Researchers, Inc.

comparison to a bacterium, a virus could be viewed as being atomic. We tend to think of a colony of bacteria as having a personality of its own, a distinct entityness, if you will. A virus is much more like a mutating atom, without a particular personality, or, perhaps more appropriately, with a personality that is always changing. It is as if the nature of a virus mutates atomically in the presence of any living field and takes on that personality. If this is so, the more certain it becomes that change and the need for change is what the virus is trying to "teach" us.

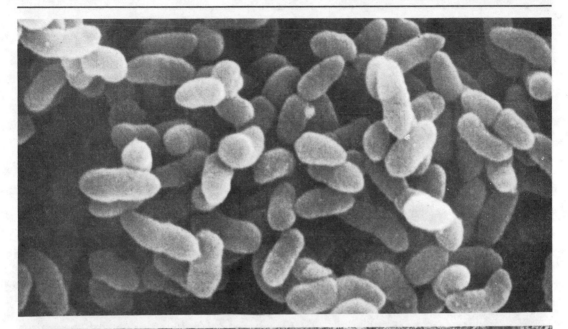

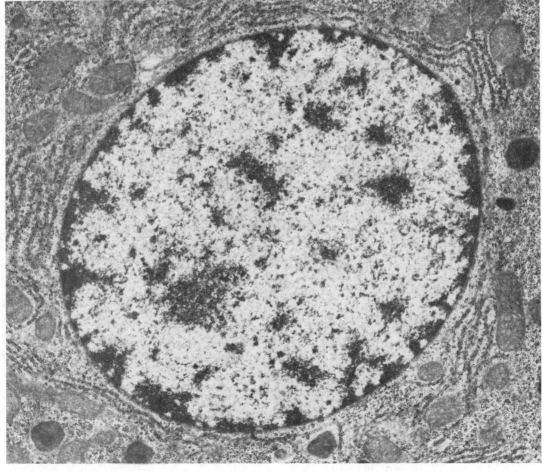

243

Listening to the Kundalini

The process of life, the path to consciousness begins with the physical body. We cannot "know" anything until we sense it or experience it first. Personal choices and decisions should "arise" from the kundalini. But since our bodies are usually quite numb, this can be a long, slow process.

One must begin to look for friends, teachers and mates by the quality of their light, not by the way they look, not by the way they say they are, but by the way the body feels in presence with them. We often choose our friends and our loved ones and proximity to them for all the wrong reasons. Many of us come from a background in which our parents did not carry a lot of light or carried light at times that was harmful to us in some way. As a result we respond to people who have abundant energy as people to be avoided, and we sense people with low energies as being safe. Such responses do not assist us to lead the powerful kind of lives that most of us desire. The kundalini has a story to tell us. We must as individuals and as a culture learn to listen to it: it is the story of life itself.

The one constant theme in that story of life is change. Gone are the days when we could believe that "nothing changes". To the contrary, the lesson of modern times is that there is nothing which does *not* change— politically, socially, individually or cellularly. The challenge which presents itself in this New Age is to both *accept* and to *control* change. On a cellular level we know that uncontrolled change can create a deadly cancer, while a *failure* to change inevitably leads to atrophy and most certain death as well. It is only in *controlling change* by consciously reorganizing our lives and moving toward those elements which carry light that we can hope to strengthen ourselves and defend against devastating disease. It is only in that conscious choice both to accept and control change that we can begin to evolve in the presence of all that makes us whole, and consciously choose to evolve toward wholeness itself. These must be the considerations of every healer in the treatment of disease. They must as well be the considerations of everyone who hopes to maintain a strong energy system capable of meeting the challenges of a constantly changing planet and an evolving consciousness.

APPENDIX
The Rolf Study

excerpted from

PROJECT REPORT:
A STUDY OF STRUCTURAL INTEGRATION FROM NEUROMUSCULAR, ENERGY FIELD, AND EMOTIONAL APPROACHES

Chapter VI. Energy Field Studies
Electronic Aura Study

by

Valerie V. Hunt, Ed.D.

The rationale and procedures used in this study to obtain electronic recordings of the auric fields came from four separate pilot studies and a prior SI [structural integration] study using EMG equipment.

Data taken from muscle during four rolfing sessions showed a changing baseline in different body areas during pain, emotional experiences and memory flash-backs with steady low voltage wave forms that did not resemble muscle depolarization. Experienced meditators after several minutes meditation and a dancer who reported reaching an altered state of consciousness displayed similar patterns.

These same low millivoltage signals were obtained from the chakra areas of a subject undergoing "Auric treatment" by a shaman healer who moved and chanted around the reclining subject. During treatment Rosalyn Bruyere, a nationally recognized aura reader, recorded the changes in shape and movement in the field. Analysis of these data disclosed that the sound, the specific acts, and the quality of the shaman's movement appeared to have no direct relation to the spurts of activity, its location or pattern. However, there was a direct correspondence between the report of the aura reader and the electronic recordings. . . .

Procedures

Continuous electronic auric field recordings were collected from four experimental subjects, Group II, during each of the ten SI sessions.

Silver/silver chloride bipolar electrodes affixed by double adhesive discs were placed on the skin over major chakra and acupuncture locations. Data were intercepted by a four channel Signatron Model 4200 FM telemetry EMG instrument, IRIG channels 11, 12, 13, 14 and a twenty thousand cycle carrier band high frequency channel and recorded on track one of a two track Nagra III tape recorder. Simultaneously with the electronic data, Rosalyn Bruyere recorded a running report of the color, size and energy movement of the chakras and auric cloud of the subject and the auric fields of the rolfers on track two, the audio track. Using a second microphone, subjects were able to describe their spontaneous experiences, images and feeling states during rolfing. The project director monitored all incoming audio and electronic data by earphones and two oscilloscopes located in a glass enclosed instrument room, and was in direct communication with the aura reader by a separate audio system. In this way she could question the aura reader about changes in the electrical signal and slate on the data tape any important information observed in the data or experimental situation. No clues about wave shape changes were ever reported to the aura reader during recording. . . .

General Findings

By the second session clearly defined wave forms were recognizable when the aura reader described different colors in chakra locations. This was such an amazing observation that if the wave form changed in any chakra and the aura reader had not reported color change she was questioned. After the wave forms were recognizable, there was direct correspondence in every instance throughout all the recordings between these wave forms and the "reader's" description of primary and secondary colors in the specific chakras. However, no discriminating wave forms were ever recognized for color blends such as mauve, turquoise or apricot. Once when all recordings dropped so low in amplitude as to be suspect, the "reader" described that the auric field had moved six feet away from and not in contact with the body. . . .

Specific findings from the electronic data and auric readings are:

1. There was a progressive improvement of energy flow upward during the ten sessions. During the early sessions the chakras were uneven, small, low in frequency and amplitude, with indiscriminate or dark primary colors. In later sessions the chakras became even in size, light in color with high amplitude, high frequency wave forms. Some chakras were closed during the early sessions with negligible recordings. As these opened the chakras showed a kaleidoscope of colors: dark blue, yellow, red orange and olive green. The "reader" described a central vertical internal flow prior to the auric changes.

The second hour more energy appeared in the legs with an increase in both chakra and aura activity. During sessions one through three the "reader" frequently reported mixed downward color displacement with the kundalini area a dark brown, the throat purple or the knee yellow. By the fifth hour all subjects had a clear blue aura. The "reader" likened this to the field of a creative person manifesting.

During the fifth and sixth hour one subject produced a secondary pink aura five to ten feet wide. The amplitude of the electronic recordings dropped but maintained a steady blue wave form. The subject appeared quiet and in great peace. The "reader" stated the subject was in an altered consciousness. During the seventh and eighth sessions there was a preponderance of light blended colors: pink, peach, ice blue and cream. As subjects reported pleasant effects, the data contained higher frequencies.

A cream colored aura appeared on all subjects during the eighth session, maintained throughout the ninth and tenth hour and was evident between sessions and during the post testing one week later.

Despite the similar overall change there were persistent individual chakra patterns evident from the first session. For example, the physiological psychologist and meditator showed greatest activity in the throat and third eye, the dancer in the feet and legs, the actress in the heart, kundalini and caduceus locations and the artist in the crown chakra.

2. Chakras frequently carried the color stated in metaphysical literature, such as red kundalini, orange hypogastric or emotional body, yellow spleen, green heart, blue throat, violet third eye, and white crown, although this was not always the case. The energy dynamically moved up and down the body with a downward placement of chakra colors in the early sessions and an upward displacement in the later sessions. . . .

3. Certain chakras seemed to be directly related. Increased activity of the kundalini, red, triggered the throat chakra, blue, while activation of the hypogastric or emotional body, orange, showed linkage with the third eye, violet. The heart and throat chakras were consistently the most active. When subjects expressed anxiety, amplitude elevated in these areas. . . .

4. Subjects had numerous emotional experiences, images and memory recall when rolfers were working on different areas verifying Reich's beliefs that memory of experiences are stored in body tissue. Furthermore, chakra activity seemed to relate to imagery content. For example, both men and women reported images of men when their right leg was rolfed; the left leg brought experiences with women. Such is in line with the concepts of the male and female aspects of the body expressed in the Chinese yin and yang, and the Jungian animus and anima. In different sessions four subjects showed a sudden high frequency and amplitude violet-purple wave form shifting from the third eye to throat and back to the third eye just prior to imaging or picturing. It is noteworthy that such a reversal pattern occurred only in the throat and third eye and always as a forerunner to imaging. (During these instances) the "reader" reported the central vertical flow decreased, the crown chakra plumed, and a secondary bubble of purple-orchid formed five feet away. . . .

5. Ordinarily rolfers' hands and arms carried a large blue or white corona with only minor changes during the sessions. When subjects expressed pain, some of their chakras recorded red, while the rolfer's aura suddenly changed to violet-pink, calming the field. The violet-pink aura has been likened to spiritual, empathetic and loving states.

After the first few sessions, subjects seemed less affected by pain; red was absent from their auric fields, and muscular responses lessened. They seemed to flow with the pain as they accepted the soothing violet of the rolfers. When subjects reported higher consciousness states or imaging, the rolfers' auras were pure white. Memory recall of early life experiences occurred with all subjects during sessions with one rolfer. . . .

Wave Forms

As raw data from chakras was monitored during each session with oscilloscopes and loud speakers, continuous wave trains were noted to contain distinct characteristics and sounds that in concert with the "reader's" reports could be described by a pure color. Oscilloscope settings were in the low 0-30 millivoltages with a sweep speed of from 5 to 50 milliseconds per centimeter based on the frequencies of the wave form.

The following reproductions of pure color wave forms ["A" in figures below] were made using a Biomation Transient Recorder No. 802 to store the wave form and expand and project it on an oscilloscope for photography. Settings on the transient recorder were selected to give the best representation of the wave details rather than with an attempt to capture specific frequency information.

Primary colors had the most distinctive patterns. Blends and light colors produced irregular, inconsistent patterns. Secondary colors contained less distinct form but nonetheless showed discriminating characteristics.

Frequency Analysis

[To determine the variety of frequencies within each of the wave forms], raw data samples of these . . . were further processed by Fourier analysis using a . . . Spectrum Analyzer. . . .

Because most of the frequencies of these data were found to lie between 110 Hz and 1000 Hz the frequency setting of the Spectrum Analyzer was at 100 Hz displayed on the X or horizontal scale of the scope. . . . However [it is possible] the carrier frequencies of the five telemetry channels at 7,350 Hz, 10,500 Hz, 14,500 Hz, 20,000 Hz and 22,000 Hz may have interfered with [the] higher frequency recordings. With more refined instruments and processing techniques the chakra energies may be found to lie also in the higher KiloHertz range[s].

From frequency analysis of many of the samples distinct frequency bands were discovered for each color irrespective of chakras. These bands were considerably lower in frequencies than those of the light spectrum.

As can be seen in the [following frequency analysis] Figures, each color contained all frequencies from 100 Hz to 1000 Hz. It was the larger quantity of energy lying at one level of the broad band (or from 10 to 20 dB above other frequencies) which differentiated the colors. Note that the primary colors showed a wider band width than the secondary colors.

Frequency analyses of energies described as secondary colors showed narrower bands lying between and slightly overlapping primary colors. As secondary color wave forms blended so did the frequency spectra.

[Oscilloscope and Spectrum Analyzer Printouts]

Figure 1. Primary Color Red

Red [*wave form*] had large sharp clumps of regular and irregular positive and negative spikes of short duration interspersed with plateaus containing small, high frequency spikes (Figure 1A). The sound resembled the high whine of a siren.

Red showed a broad *frequency* band between 640 and 800 Hz that merged with orange in the lower frequencies and with upper blue in the higher ones (Figure 1B). The onset of red waves was distinctly related to subjects' expression of pain by sounds and muscular agitation. In this experiment red frequencies were short lived. When rolfing was discontinued momentarily, the red wave shifted back and forth to orange, as though emotional processing was still going on. The literature describes red auric fields related to strong pure natural emotional states, to physical vitality or life force and to instinctual energies. From these and other auric observations we postulated that the experience of pain may cause an alarm reaction activating the red frequencies or life force.

A. Red Wave Form **B. Fourier Frequency Analysis**

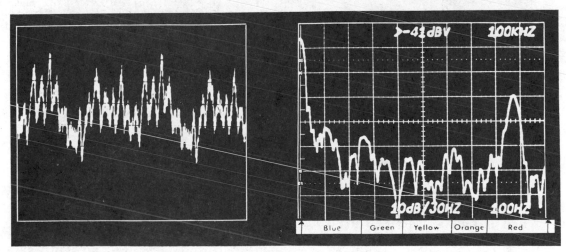

Figure 2. Secondary Color Orange

Orange [*wave form*] showed sharp peaks of short equal duration, low amplitude interspersed with sharp peaks of longer duration and higher amplitude. It resembled red in the sharpness of the peaks with lower amplitude plateaus. It contained some regularity of yellow but was faster and without the small overlaying spikes. It differed from violet in the longer duration of large peaks and contained no saw tooth effect (Figure 4). It was lower in tone than the red and contained some of the wandering tonal qualities of yellow.

Orange wave forms derived from auric readings showed a narrow *frequency* band between yellow and red at 600 Hz to 740 Hz (Figure 2B). The raw wave forms also resembled red and yellow. Again the incidences were limited primarily to one subject who had longer periods of emotional expression, weeping, flailing and clenching fists that seemed to accompany great pain and intense imagery. There is common agreement in the literature linking orange auric fields to emotional states.

A. Orange Wave Form　　　　　　**B. Fourier Frequency Analysis**

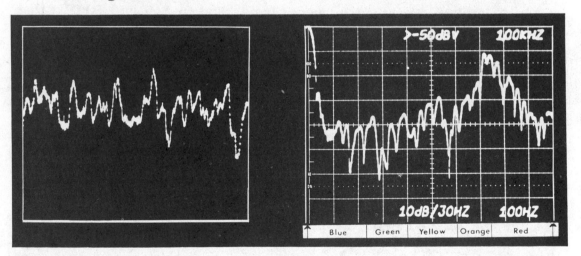

Figure 3. Primary Color Yellow

Yellow [*wave form*] showed a broad smooth wave resembling an uneven sine wave with an occasional slow rounded peak. Smaller irregular positive and negative deflections overlayed the entire wave form (Figure 3A). Wandering musical tones were characteristic of the sound.

Yellow contained *frequencies* from 400 Hz to 600 Hz (Figure 3B). Although yellow was not a prevalent color in this study, at times all chakras recorded a preponderance of these frequencies. This color occurred most often when subjects described a strong will to overcome pain or in intellectually coping with frustration. Metaphysical literature describes the yellow aura related to the intellectual phase of mentality, to logical reasoning and synthesis.

A. Yellow Wave Form   **B. Fourier Frequency Analysis**

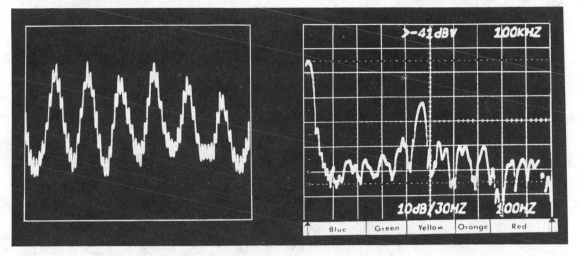

Figure 4. Secondary Color Green

Green [*wave form*] had the overall characteristics of a broad uneven sine wave of yellow yet with more irregular sharper deflections containing double peaks like the blue. Characteristic of yellow, slight spikings overlayed the major waves (Figure 4A). The wandering musical tones of yellow were combined with the rolling rumble of blue.

Green *frequencies* between 240 and 400 Hz were infrequent in these subjects during rolfing (Figure 4B). However, other pilot studies supplied sufficient data to verify the band spectrum. The raw wave form had characteristics of both yellow and blue and likewise the frequency band of green lay between these two colors. Green has been attributed to transition . . . . In this study no clear-cut relationships emerged.

A. Green Wave Form   **B. Fourier Frequency Analysis**

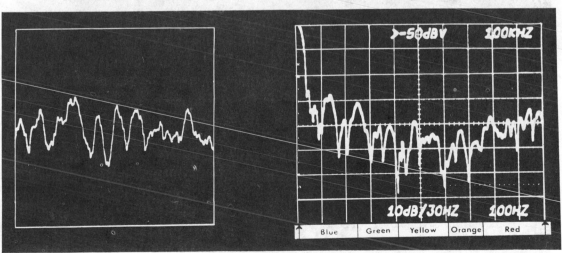

Figure 5. Primary Color Blue

Blue [*wave form*] showed medium large, sharp positive and negative deflections with single or double peaks at the top of the deflection. The broad ascending and descending slopes of the major deflections contained small saw-tooth peaks (Figure 5A). The sound was an irregular rumble.

Blue, the most prevalent color, produced two *frequency* bands with a preponderance in the lower band from 100 Hz to 240 Hz and a narrower upper band around 800 Hz (Figure 5B). This was a continuous wave form that did not resemble the on and off quality of muscle depolarization and was lower in amplitude, yet it still contained frequencies from 100 Hz - 200 Hz characteristic of motor unit action. Combined with the fact that the lower frequency band was out of sequence with the light spectrum, we speculated that it must arise from small high frequency motor units or muscle spindles. The large slow spikes and the small saw-tooth spikes noted in the raw wave forms possibly represent these two frequency bands. All other color frequencies as well as the upper band of blue were considerably above frequencies from muscle recordings [taken] from surface electrodes leading us to postulate a different energy source, possibly cellular or subatomic as described in the physics literature.

A. Blue Wave Form   **B. Fourier Frequency Analysis**

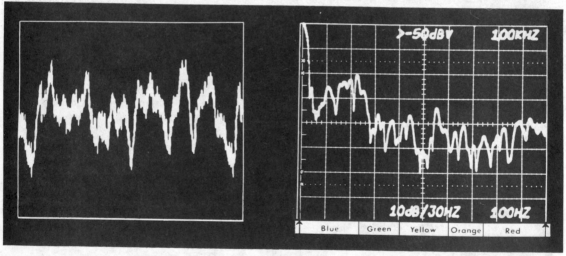

Figure 6. Secondary Color Violet-Purple

Violet-Purple [*wave form*] contained short, rapid sharp spikes of approximately equal duration but varying in amplitude with occasional small plateaus like red and smaller less defined saw-tooth effect resembling the blue form (Figure 6A). The low background rumble of blue was overlayed by the higher red siren sound.

The secondary color purple was rarely described by the aura reader. Instead, shades of violet, orchid and indigo were most often seen. The reader explained that purple contained many of the high frequencies of white and therefore appeared in lighter shades. The purple shades customarily found in the middle and later sessions carried a narrow *frequency* band at about 900 Hz (Figure 6B). The spectrum analysis also showed about equal high peakings at 100 - 200 Hz, blue and 740 - 900 Hz, red, as the purple shade wave forms also contained these color characteristics. Violet has been likened to a high consciousness state associated with the creative or spiritual mode.

A. Violet-Purple Wave Form   **B. Fourier Frequency Analysis**

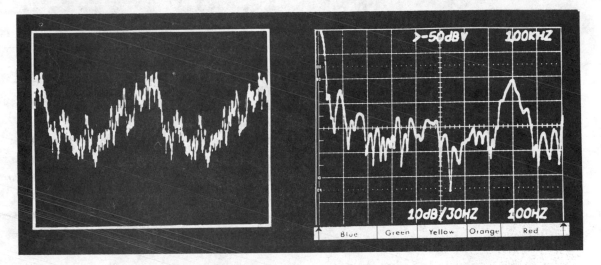

Figure 7. Primary Color White

White [*wave form*] appeared to resemble white noise with such short high amplitude positive and negative spikes as to obliterate any other wave shape. When processed through a transient recorder the high spikes of the blue, the hash of yellow and plateaus of red become evident. These characteristics were not noted in the raw data (Figure 7A). The sound of white was distinctive yet difficult to describe. It had a similar high pitch to white noise but the random quality of noise was interrupted at times with the rumble, the tones and the scream of blue, yellow and red.

The spectrum analysis of the white wave form gave almost symmetrically equal *frequencies* throughout the entire spectrum from 100 Hz to 1000 Hz with no evidence of distinct color bands (Figure 7B). [Differentials] were five decibels or less. There appeared a concave ascending amplitude curve with slightly smaller amounts of the 300 Hz to 600 Hz or the green and orange spectra, and slightly larger amounts of the blue, yellow, red and violet spectra. Random incidences occurred throughout the ten sessions except with one subject who often produced white when he catapulted into an altered state during pain or uncomfortable imagery. Other subjects produced a white aura and/or white pluming from the crown chakra associated with "out of body" experiences. White auric emissions have been associated with the highest level of consciousness or mind, and with the spirit, accompanied by changes in ordinary reality.

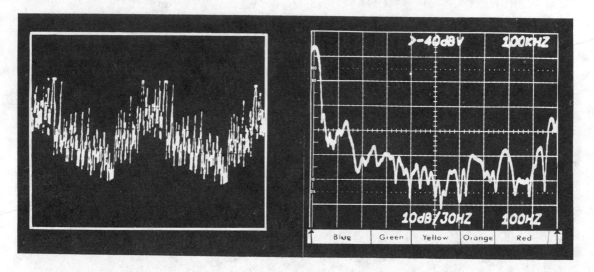

A. White Wave Form **B. Fourier Frequency Analysis**

Figure 8. Secondary Color Cream

Cream color [*wave form*] in the raw data could not be differentiated from white. . . . [Detailed analyses] showed the same high frequency spiking of white yet with [fewer] broad blue spikes and more of the hash spikings and plateaus characteristic of yellow and red. The sound likewise resembled the white.

The aura reader described a prevalent cream colored aura beginning with the eighth session. She reported she had never before seen this auric color nor has it been reported in the literature. The raw wave form resembled white in sharp high *frequency* spikings but with no other discriminating characteristics. The spectrum analyses showed slightly less symmetrical frequencies from 100 Hz to 1000 Hz like white yet with a bit less amplitude in the 800 Hz to 900 Hz bands of blue and violet, and slightly greater amplitude in the 500 Hz to 800 Hz bands of red and yellow (Figure 8B). How long this color frequency pattern continued is not yet known. It did persist during and between the last three sessions, at post testing, and has been observed by the "reader" in rolfed subjects several months later. There are no definite clues to indicate whether the cream color often produced by these rolfed subjects is an artificial field resulting from some systemic reaction to connective tissue manipulation; whether it represents a modulated active life force with an alert sensory processing system of a refined high level consciousness or results from unknown reasons carrying other meanings. Further energy field and physiological studies may elucidate this finding.

A. Cream Wave Form

B. Fourier Frequency Analysis

Not
Available

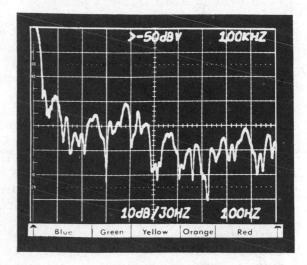

Sonogram Frequency Analysis

In an attempt to obtain more detail relative to the aura reader's elaborate reports, the same data loops that produced the wave forms and spectrum frequency bands were further processed by an Audio Spectrum Analyzer. [For additional information regarding this part of the study, the actual "Rolf Study" can be consulted. Write the Rolf Institute for further information or watch for Dr. Hunt's forthcoming book, described at the end of this Appendix.]

Conclusion

What do these detailed findings mean? The possible interpretations are staggering. These data constitute radiations taken directly from the body surface, quantitatively measured in a natural state containing frequencies and patterns that were isolated by scientifically accepted data reduction procedures. Three different data resolutions by wave form, by Fourier frequency analysis and by Sonogram frequency representation all produced the same results, differing only in the fineness of definition. Furthermore these findings taken from chakra locations were in direct correspondence with the aura reader's description of chakra energy and frequently depicted the total auric cloud. Throughout the centuries in which sensitives have seen and described the auric emissions, this is the first objective electronic evidence of frequency, amplitude and time which validates their subjective observation of color discharge.

257

The fact that these discovered color frequencies do not duplicate those of light or pigment does not negate the finding. When we realize that what we see as colors are frequencies picked up by the eye, differentiated and allotted a word symbol, then there is nothing to indicate that the eye and the brain processing centers interpret color only in the high kilohertz frequencies. The ultimate criterion for the experience of color is the visual interpretation of frequency representation. However, with finer instruments, improved recording and data reduction techniques, these data now primarily up to 1500 Hz may very readily contain much higher frequencies.

This study discovered energy emanations from the body surface beyond frequencies here-to-fore found coming from biochemical systems. At the present time these findings can be interpreted only by an energy field conceptual model.

Further, the study discloses that rolfing is a powerful modality to alter this field toward more refined equal and higher frequencies. The tremendous detail described by the aura reader throughout 60 hours of rolfing concerning the individual auric responses, group reactions to sessions and the relationship between emotional states and auric color should be viewed as facts and not subjective judgments. Many of the continuously expressed experiences of subjects during SI [structural integration] carry such dynamic corollary changes in the energy field that these cannot be minimized.

From the extensive detailed study of energy field emissions from the body meticulously recorded and processed, strong conclusions are warranted. The energy field described as aura has dynamic changes that coincide with emotional states, imagery, interpersonal relations and the state of resiliency and plasticity of the connective tissue of the physical body. A skilled aura reader can accurately describe the color and dynamic interplay of this electromagnetic energy radiating from chakras and forming the auric field. And finally SI [structural integration] makes consistent and progressive changes in the auric emissions based upon areas of the body processed during each session. The end results were a uniformly higher frequency, more coherent energy field for all four subjects studied. The widespread implications for psychophysical health are profound.

Furthermore the extensive ramifications for further study of health, disease, pain, psychopathology and all human behavior using the techniques discovered in this study are beyond estimation.

NOTE: This report has been slightly rearranged from the original to produce a document easier for non-technical minds to follow. The essence of the report is not lost by these changes. And wording of the original was left entirely in tact (except where noted).

MIND FIELDS: THE SCIENCE OF HUMAN VIBRATIONS
by Dr. Valerie Hunt

expands this information and presents an energy field model of bio-cosmic interface and the emotional, mystical happenings which lead to healing responses, spiritual experiences and evolution.

This unique work culminates eighteen years of electronic laboratory and clinical research into relationships between biological phenomena and Mind Fields. The research reveals sources of great depth and connects these fields to consciousness, allowing new scientific explanations. Such understanding provides clear directions for the individual achievement of emotional freedom, spiritual strength and health.

GLOSSARY
Volume 1

Alternating Current (AC): An electric current that reverses its direction at regular recurring intervals.

Alzheimer's Disease: A disease evidenced by a slow, continuous decline in intellectual function due to atrophy of frontal and occipital lobes. Memory, speech and gait are also often affected as a result.

Amplitude: The extent of a vibratory movement (as of a pendulum) measured from a mean position to an extreme; the maximum departure of the value of an alternating current or wave from the average value.

Androgynous: Having characteristics or the nature of both male and female.

Archetype: The original pattern of which all things of the same type are representations; also an inherited idea or mode of thought in the psychology of C.G. Jung that is derived from the experience of the race and is present in the unconscious of the individual.

Astral Plane: That level or realm of consciousness which bridges the dimensions of matter and spirit; the plane in which we dream; the body of the fourth chakra.

Atman: One of the two higher chakras that exist outside the body.

Aura: A luminous radiation which emanates from all living matter; a distinctive atmosphere surrounding a given source; also a subtle sensory stimulus.

Auric Field: The electromagnetic field which emanates from all matter.

Axon: The long thin portion of a nerve cell that as a rule conducts impulses away from the cell body. Impulses move from dendrite to cell body and cell body to synapse.

Biofeedback: The technique of making unconscious or involuntary bodily processes (as heartbeat or brain waves) perceptive to the senses (as by the use of an oscilloscope) in order to manipulate them by conscious mental control.

Blocked Chakra: One in which energy flow has been somehow restricted.

Bodhisattva: One who compassionately refrains from entering nirvana (state of oblivion) in order to assist others on their evolutionary journey.

Brahman Gate: (Hindu) Name given to the seventh chakra, located at the top of the head.

Brahman: Second of the two higher chakras existing outside the body.

Candidiasis: A yeast infection produced by the yeastlike fungus *candida albicans* which is a common inhabitant of the mouth, vagina, and intestinal tract.

Celestial Plane: The realm of pure light, visualization and archetype; the body of the sixth chakra.

Chakra: (Sanskrit) Wheel of light; one of the energy centers within the body, the spinning of which generates an electromagnetic or auric field around the body.

Chakra Body: An area of existing or potential consciousness that dictates a particular attitude toward reality. There are seven major chakra bodies: physical, emotional, mental, astral, etheric, celestial, ketheric.

Chakra Harmonics: Varying frequency bands of the same color or wave form.

Chakra Openness: Capacity of any given chakra which allows for energy flow within or through a chakra.

Chakra Intensity: Amount of energy produced by a particular chakra.

Channeling: A term used to describe the healing technique in which one person (the healer) acts as a channel to transfer various frequencies of energy to another person (the client) for the purpose of rebalancing chakras (stabilizing the electromagnetic field), thereby facilitating stress reduction, regeneration of tissues and healing.

Chelation: A process of clearing and charging the aura in which energy is channeled into the client's body in progressive steps beginning at the feet and moving up the body and the chakra system.

Circadian Rhythm: The prevailing biological cycle of all living things.

Clairaudience: The ability to hear sound beyond the range of normal hearing.

Clairsentience: Responsive to or conscious of sense perceptions and feelings at a level beyond normal perception.

Clairvoyance: The ability to perceive matters or images beyond the range of normal perception including subtle body energies, chakras and auric fields.

Closed Chakra: See "blocked chakra".

Colitis: Inflammation of the colon.

Connective Tissue: That tissue which pervades, supports and binds together other tissues and forms ligaments, tendons and aponeuroses; a tissue of mesodermal origin rich in intercellular substance or interlacing processes with little tendency for the cells to come together in sheets or masses.

Dedifferentiation: Reversion of cells or other specialized structures to a more generalized or primitive condition often as a preliminary to major change.

Dendrite: The end of a nerve cell that receives the message, impulse or stimulus and carries it toward the cell body.

Differentiation: Development from the one to the many, the simple to the complex or the homogeneous to the heterogeneous; cell modification of body parts so a particular cell can perform its intended particular functions; the sum of the processes whereby apparently indifferent cells, tissues and structures attain their adult form and function.

Direct Current (DC): An electric current flowing in one direction only and substantially constant in value.

Down's Syndrome: The preferred term for mongolism, a variety of congenital moderate-to-severe mental retardation.

Dynamic Field: An electromagnetic field in which a disturbance has caused a wave form to be emitted and thus a time varying electric and magnetic field to form.

Electrical Charge: A quantity of electricity resulting from the random motion of electrons residing on the surface of an electrified body. Electrons have a negative charge (by definition); thus a negatively charged body has an excess of electrons; a positively charged body has a shortage of electrons. An electric current flowing through a conductor changes the random movement to an orderly drifting.

Electrical Field Potential: The relative voltage at a point in an electric circuit or field with respect to some reference point in the same circuit or field. Voltage, which can exist without a current, can potentially cause a current to flow when a circuit is closed.

Electric Current: A movement of electrons analogous to the flow of a stream. By means of a conductor, free electrons are guided in an orderly fashion from a negatively charged body to a positively charged one.

Electrode: A conductor used to establish electrical contact with a nonmetallic part of a circuit.

Electrolyte: A nonmetallic electric conductor in which current is carried by movement of ions; a substance which when dissolved in a suitable solvent or when fused becomes an ionic conductor.

Electromagnetic Field: The space around a charged object where an electric field exists in a perpendicular direction to a magnetic field.

Electromagnetism: Magnetism developed by a current of electricity; a branch of physical science that deals with the physical relationship between electricity and magnetism.

Empirical: Relying on experience or observation alone often without due regard for system and theory; originating in or based on observation or experience; capable of being verified or disproved by observation or experiment.

Energy: The capacity for doing work or the capacity for action or being active; also, natural power vigorously exerted.

Etheric Plane: Realm of pure sound and pure thought void of light; the spiritual template for the physical world; the body of the fifth chakra.

Exogenous: Originating from or due to external causes.

Fascia: A sheet of connective tissue covering or binding together body structures. It encloses and wraps all muscles, organs and bones.

Feminine Chakra: One which attracts or pulls; one of negative polarity; an intake chakra; namely, the second, fourth and sixth.

Frequency: The number of repetitions of a periodic process in a unit of time as (a) the number of complete alterations per second of an alternating current, (b) the number of sound waves per second produced by a sounding body, and (c) the number of complete oscillations per second of an electromagnetic wave.

Glia: A cell of neuroglia, having many branches; a tissue composed of a variety of cells, mostly glial cells, that makes up most of the nervous system.

Hedonistic: In agreement with the doctrine that pleasure or happiness is the chief good in life.

Hermetic Tradition: Relating to the teachings or writings attributed to Hermes Trismegistus, legendary author of works embodying magical, astrological and alchemical doctrines.

Hertz: A unit of frequency equal to the cycle per second.

Intake Chakra: One into which energy flows; a chakra of negative polarity; namely, the second, fourth and sixth.

Kachina: The spiritual components of the outer physical forms of life, which may be invoked to manifest their benign powers so man may be enabled to continue his evolutionary journey; also, inner forms and respected spirits among Indians of the Southwest, specifically the Hopi.

Kether: From the Hebrew, meaning "crown", the Highest of the Ten Sephiroth in the Kabbala.

Ketheric Plane: Realm of pure energy and spirit and mergence with Deity; the body of the seventh chakra.

Kinesiology: The study of the principle of mechanics and anatomy in relation to human movement.

Kinetic: Of, or relating to the motion of material bodies and the forces and energy associated therewith.

Kinetic Energy: Energy associated with motion, in contrast to potential energy which is energy in storage.

Kirlian Photography: A method of capturing on a photographic plate an image of what is purported to be an aura of energy that emanates from animals and plants and that undergoes changes in accordance with physiological or emotional changes.

Kiva: A Pueblo Indian (mainly Hopi and Zuni) ceremonial structure.

Kundalini: The awakened or sleeping "Serpent Power" located in the first chakra.

Magnitude: A number given to a quantity for purposes of comparison with other quantities of the same class.

Medicine Stories: In the Native American tradition, stories told intended to connect the listener to some sacred inner wisdom.

Mysteries: Secret rites or doctrines known only to a small, esoteric group; specifically in ancient Greece, religious ceremonies or doctrines revealed only to the initiated; also, any of the ancient cults characterized by such ceremonies, as the Eleusinian Mysteries.

Magnetism: A class of physical phenomena believed to be inseparably associated with moving electricity exhibited by both magnets and electric currents, and characterized by fields of force.

Masculine Chakra: One which pushes energy out or through the system; one of positive polarity; an output chakra.

Mind Field: A concept which refers to the mind as an electromagnetic or energy field as opposed to a brain-centered definition.

Nerve Plexus: A network of interlacing nerves.

Neuron: A grayish or reddish granular cell with specialized processes that is the fundamental functional unit of nervous tissue.

Neurotransmitter: A naturally produced body chemical used to carry the nerve impulse across the synapse (q.v.).

Ontogeny: The division or course of division of an individual organism.

Open Chakra: A chakra through which energy flows properly and freely.

Oracle: The place of prophecy, the prophet and the prophecy itself.

Oscillation: The action of variation or fluctuation; a flow of electricity changing periodically from a maximum to a minimum; a single swing (as an oscillating body) from one extreme to the other.

Output Chakra: One which moves energy out the front of the body; a chakra of positive polarity; namely, the first, third, fifth and seventh chakras.

Perineural: Relating to the perineurium (q.v.).

Perineurium: The connective-tissue sheath that surrounds a bundle of nerve fibers.

Periosteum: The membrane of connective tissue that closely invests all bones except at the articular surfaces.

Phylogeny: The evolution of a genetically related group of organisms as distinguished from the division of the individual organism.

Piezoelectricity: Electrical current generated by repeated mechanical bending or deformations of certain crystals such as germanium and silicon.

Polarity: The property possessed by bodies having opposite magnetic poles of placing themselves so that their two extremities point to the two magnetic poles of the earth; any tendency to turn, grow, think, feel, etc, in a certain way or direction, as if because of magnetic attraction or repulsion; the condition of being positive or negative with respect to some reference point or object.

Potential: Something that can develop or become actual; any of the various functions from which the intensity or the velocity at any point in a field may be readily calculated; specif.: the degree of electrification as referred to some standard; another term for voltage, which may at times exist without a current but is potentially able to cause a current to flow, once a circuit is completed.

Potential Energy: Energy that is the result of relative position instead of motion, as in a coiled spring. It is also energy in storage waiting to be exerted.

Prana: (Also known as chi or ki) The name given to the vital life force or energy in the body, accessible through breath.

Primary Auric Field: The inner shell of the aura, generated by the spinning of the first, third and fifth chakras.

Propagation: The extension or transmission (esp. sound waves or electro-magnetic radiation) through air or water.

Pyroelectricity: Electrical current generated by the heating of certain crystals.

Redifferentiation: The process in which a previously mature cell which has dedifferentiated becomes a mature, specialized cell once more.

Rolfing: Name commonly given to Structural Integration, a system of reshaping and realigning body posture through deep (and sometimes painful) stretching of the muscle fascia accomplished by direct, deep manipulation.

Scanning: A healing technique in which the healer moves his or her hand over the edges of the client's aura in an attempt to obtain necessary information about energy flow.

Schwann Cells: Cells which surround all of the nerves outside of the brain and spinal cord. They wrap around larger axons of peripheral nerves to form multilayered myelin sheaths.

Sciatic Nerve: Of, relating to, or situated near the hip; the main nerve from the lower back that extends down into the leg.

Second Sight: The capacity to see auras, chakras, energy fields as well as remote, past or future objects or events.

Secondary Auric Field: The outer shell of the aura, produced from the interaction of all seven major chakras.

Semiconductor:: A substance, as germanium or silicon, whose conductivity is poor at low temperatures but is improved by minute additions of certain substances or by the application of heat, light or voltage: used in transistors, rectifiers, etc. Semiconduction occurs within energy as a result of the specific crystalline molecular structure.

Shaman: A priest who uses ritual and ceremony to cure the sick, to divine the hidden and to influence events.

Sickle-cell Anemia: A disease which occurs mainly in the Black race and is caused by abnormal hemoglobin (hemoglobin S, or Hb S), that is sensitive to oxygen deficiency.

Siddhi Powers: Those usually acquired through the mastery of the higher stages of yoga. "Siddhi" means "perfection" in Hindu. Clairvoyance, clairsentience, clairaudience, levitation, teleportation, bilocation and healing are examples of some siddhi powers.

Static Field: An electromagnetic field where no fluctuations are occurring and no wave forms are being emitted.

Structural Integration: See "Rolfing".

Superconductivity: An almost complete disappearance of electrical resistance in various metals at temperatures near absolute zero.

Sushumna: (Yoga) One of the main channels or nadis ("conduits", "vessels", "veins" or "nerves") of the body through which vital energy circulates. It extends from the base of the spine to the crown of the head and the path of its energy follows (approximately) the spinal column. Entwining and flowing around it are the energies of the other two major nadis, the Ida and Pengali; an opposing downward force in the rising kundalini experience.

Synapse: The junction between one nerve cell and another or between a nerve cell and some other cell.

Thousand-petaled lotus: The seventh chakra also known as the Diamond Sutra or the Diamond Lotus.

Transmitting Energy: See "channeling".

Undifferentiated: Not specialized; a term given to cells that are in an embryonic or primitive state.

Vibrations: The periodic motion of a body or wave in alternating opposite directions from the position of zero when equilibrium has been disturbed.

Vision Quest: An essential part of a young Native American Indian's initiation into adulthood. The youth is sent on a vigil involving fasting and praying in order to gain some sign of the presence and nature of his guardian spirit. Often the sign is a dream in which his guardian spirit appears to him, usually in animal form, instructs him and takes him on a visionary journey.

Voltage: Electric potential or potential difference expressed in volts.

Wave: A disturbance or variation that transfers energy progressively from point to point. This disturbance may form an elastic deformation or a variation of pressure, electric or magnetic intensity, electric potential, or temperature.

Wave Form: In physics, any of the series of advancing impulses set up by a vibration, pulsation or disturbance in air or some other medium, as in the transmission of heat, light, sound, etc.

Wavelength: The distance between corresponding points on two successive waves: In physics, the distance, measured in the direction of progression of a wave, from any given point to the next point characterized by the same phase.

Yang: Positive masculine energy.

Yin: Negative feminine energy.

Yogi: One who practices yoga.

INDEX
Volume 1